Eat, Drink and Be Merry Through Menopause

By Doneane Beckcom

Symphony
PUBLISHING

Eat, Drink and Be Merry Through Menopause

Eat, Drink and Be Merry Through Menopause

1. Health, Fitness & Dieting – Personal Health – Women's Health

2. Health, Fitness & Dieting – Women's Health - General

3. Self Help – Mid Life

E-book Version: Kindle

ISBN-13: 978-0998304601 (Symphony Publishing)
ISBN-10: 0998304603

TABLE OF CONTENTS

Eat, Drink and Be Merry Through Menopause

Learn How to Deal with Symptoms Naturally

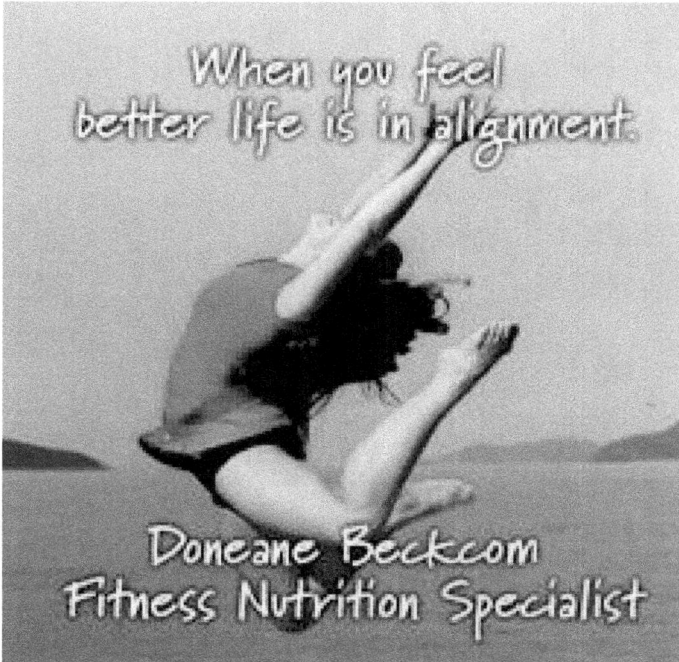

When you feel better life is in alignment.

Doneane Beckcom
Fitness Nutrition Specialist

PREFACE

Time for Change: Do something today that your future self will thank you for.

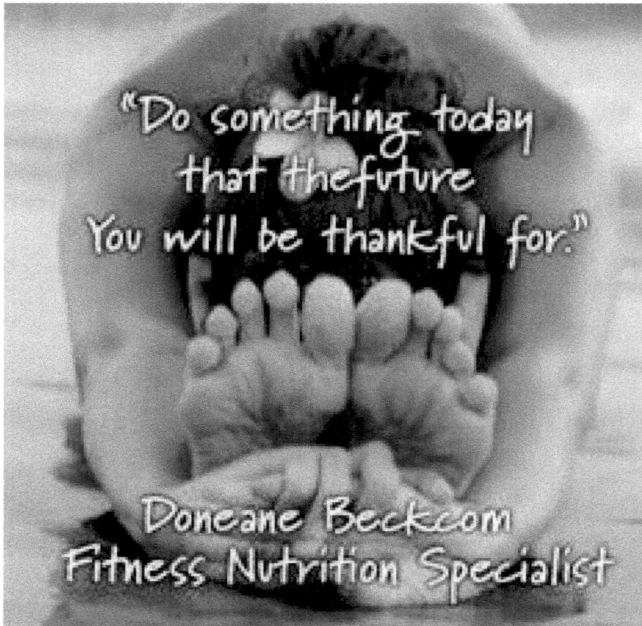

"Do something today that the future You will be thankful for."

Doneane Beck.com
Fitness Nutrition Specialist

The person I am today is very thankful for the things I did starting about 15 years ago, to get off of medications and get healthier. I can only imagine what my life would be like if I had not done that.

I am sure I would still be taking multiple medications, dealing with symptoms and pain, finding time to take my meds, go for checkups, get prescriptions filled, etc. I would not be thankful for any of that.

Where you are today is not where you were yesterday or last week. And it is not where you will be tomorrow or next week. Think about how you feel right now. I mean REALLY think about it. How did you feel when you went to bed last night? How

2

about when you woke up this morning, or first put your feet on the floor? Did you feel ready for the day and excited to get out the door for your day's activities? If you are in the midst of dealing with the symptoms of menopause, chances are you are not thinking positive thoughts about any of those questions.

But now think about this: Is that how you want to feel tomorrow, next week, next year? If the answer is no, then realize that YOU have the power to decide that it is time for things to change.

Think about where you would like to be: ten or twenty pounds lighter? Tighter, toned arms and legs? Sleeping better at night? Having more energy? Dealing with hormonal symptoms that disrupt your life?

Make a list of the things you would like to change, and then set a course for that change. Think about those things that you would like to be grateful for in a week, a month, a year from now. Heck, tomorrow! And then decide the small steps you can take to accomplish even one of those goals. You cannot do them overnight, but you CAN work on all of them daily. Each large goal can be broken down into smaller steps that can be accomplished in a logical order working toward the overall objective. This way you will not be overwhelmed and feel like you have failed.

This book is an attempt to give you the tools that you need to make healthy changes, to really DO something today that you will be thankful for down the road. I hope that, in some small way, I will give you the tools and motivation to help you feel better, restore your confidence, and allow you to experience the joy and freedom of a healthy lifestyle again.

I call menopause a "raw deal" for two reasons: (1) it can be a very raw time in life, if you are not prepared for what the symptoms can do to you; and (2) I choose to look at it from a raw standpoint – natural and without anything artificial involved, if at all possible.

I have to thank my husband for his never-ending support of ALL the things that I do, my daughter for always inspiring me to be a better Mom and person, the tribe of women in my life who have cheered me on and who know, as only women can, the hopes, dreams and yearnings of modern women – and God, for giving me the gifts and talents with which I am blessed.

Are YOU ready for the journey? LET'S GO!!!

Health & Happiness,

Doneane

Feel Better ~ Make Healthier Decisions™

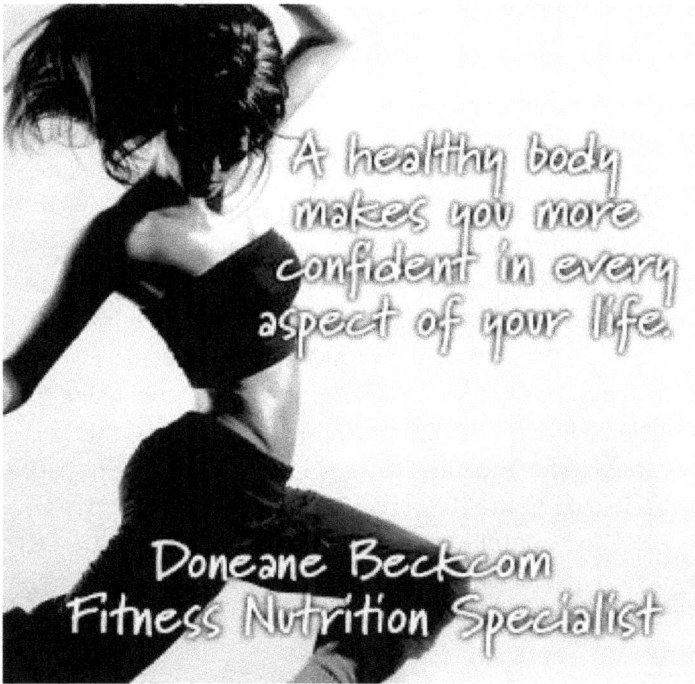

A healthy body makes you more confident in every aspect of your life.

Doneane Beckcom
Fitness Nutrition Specialist

I am Doneane Beckcom, certified nutritionist, health and wellness coach, Hatha yoga instructor, speaker and author. My passion is helping people change their eating and exercise habits so that they feel better physically, emotionally, and psychologically. When you feel better, life is in alignment and the decisions you make are better in every respect.

I have been in the fitness industry for over 30 years, starting out during the age of aerobics, ankle weights, Jane Fonda exercise videos, and unitards. As my clientele aged, my programming also aged, not because I wanted it to but because it needed to. I mean, a twentysomething doesn't want a 50-year-old trainer! And a 50-year-old shouldn't be trained by a twentysomething. In my opinion it just works better that way. I know if I was shopping for a personal trainer, I would be looking for a woman just like ME, who understands where I am in life and where I have been to get here.

So now, I am well into the not-so-wonderful stage of life that we women know as perimenopause, the period before actual menopause. I have been stuck here for about 10 years. I have had ALL of the usual symptoms – insomnia, night sweats, hot flashes, weight gain, bladder leakage, acne, lack of sex drive, heavy periods and painful cramps. It's been a rough ride! Once I went for nine months without a cycle and I was SO excited that it might really be OVER! And then BAM one day it was back with a vengeance and has not let up since. Just before publishing this book, I turned 51 so it is high time, in my opinion, that this journey comes to an end and I can say I am in actual menopause and just be DONE! In the U.S., the average age for menopausal women is 52, so hopefully I am on the downslide. I really have no way of knowing, since my mother had a total hysterectomy and oophorectomy in her late 30s and my sister is 60 and has just officially hit menopause.

GOD HELP ME if I have to do this for nine more years!!!

My gynecologist had me on low dose birth control pills for a LONG time to combat the symptoms I was experiencing, and it worked. But I grew weary of taking hormones after reading some of the doom and gloom reports about long-term effects, and decided to let my body do its thing naturally. My doctor was VERY supportive, although some are NOT. That is when my symptoms started to reappear, and they were much worse than when I first noticed them in my late 30s. I am SO thankful now that I started preparing my body for this long ago – eating clean, exercising, getting quality sleep – and I am probably much healthier because of it. Had I NOT prepared myself physically by making those changes, I can only imagine how much worse my symptoms would be.

Because I have suffered with these symptoms and have found natural remedies to combat them, I want to share this knowledge with other women, helping them to feel better – physically, emotionally, psychologically – and restore their confidence. Along the way you might even lose some weight and see some or all of those symptoms subside.

It is my goal to help you learn healthy eating habits and modify your exercise plan so that you can get your symptoms under control. When you do this, and start to feel better physically and feel good about yourself, you will make better choices in your personal and professional life. I could talk about eating habits and their impact on health and emotional issues all day, every day. I have invested thousands of dollars on nutrition and fitness training to learn as much as I can to help people like you.

For those of you at the other end of the spectrum and have passed through the dark days of symptoms, this book can still offer help. Be sure that your eating and exercise habits are such that your next decades of life can be lived in health and enjoyment and not be tied to taking daily medications.

I wasn't always so passionate about healthy eating. It was when my own health was poor and I was taking lots of meds that I took action. And I feel better now than ever. I take NO prescription medications, NO HORMONES, I go to the doctor only for required testing as I get older – and all because I took control and changed my eating and exercise habits. I rarely get "sick" to the point that I would need medical attention. Healthy food, good exercise, lots of water, sunshine, and quality sleep are my medications of choice.

My passion for good health and my love for helping others led me, in 2009, to leave the personal training business per se and launch my nutrition coaching business. I have been at the place of feeling bad and making poor life choices, not knowing where to start to make changes in life. But making better health decisions brought my life back into alignment, and allowed me to experience freedom, joy, and confidence again. I want to help you experience those same things. And while I am a big fan of "instant gratification" and the "quick fix," changing habits takes time and dedication. My approach is all about YOU! Your health is important to you – and to me.

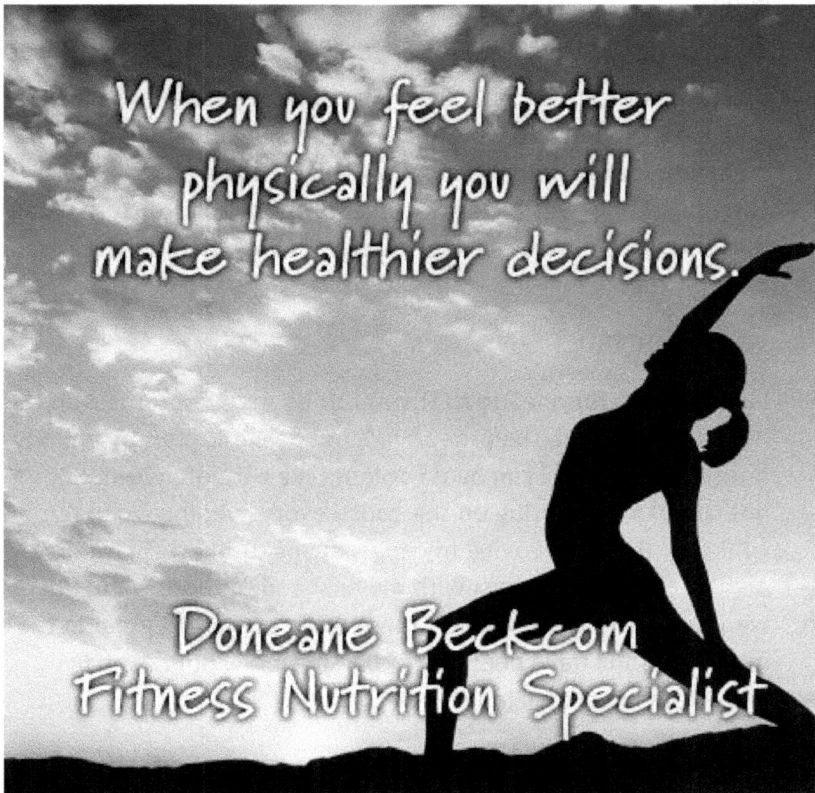

When you feel better physically you will make healthier decisions.

Doneane Beckcom
Fitness Nutrition Specialist

Think back . . . can you pinpoint when your symptoms started, when it was that you last felt good?

I mean REALLY felt good – jump-out-of- bed in the morning good, be productive during the day good, accomplish things well into the evening hours good, and getting a good night's sleep good?

I can continue this list: Not having hot flashes, night sweats, cramps and being bloated good? Not being moody, forgetful, worried about continued weight gain good? Not being concerned about how your sex life has gone down the drain good?

It's hard for me to pinpoint that exact time also. When feeling bad lasts for so many years, we get used to it; it becomes not how we feel, but who we ARE. And when we let negative talk creep into our heads, and all of our girlfriends are commiserating over the same junk, it sets us up for just thinking that this is how it is and we just have to live with it for the rest of our lives.

That is NOT TRUE!

I know that I, for one, do NOT want to be my symptoms. I do not want to be the sleep-deprived, hot flashing, crampy, moody, hormone monster I can be if I do not take care of myself. I do not want to be the slug on the couch every evening when I could be outside enjoying my dogs, my beautiful yard, a starry night, or having crazy sex with my husband for hours. I do not want to be the zombie who cannot wake up feeling great in the morning until I have been out of bed for a few hours and live with brain fog all day long.

I AM NOT THAT WOMAN!

And neither are you.

YOU DESERVE TO FEEL BETTER! YOU DESERVE TO FEEL CONFIDENT!

Dealing with menopause symptoms is an all-or-nothing proposition – you either deal with the symptoms, finding a way to help them subside, or you don't. You either start to see changes or you don't. You either begin to feel better or you don't. You cannot do it half-ass! You must embrace the process. Once you make the decision that it is time to DO something – change habits, try a new alternative treatment – you are setting on a course of CHANGE. And if you stick to it, that change can be momentous for improving your life.

And speaking of those negative Nellie girlfriends: I know you love them. I love mine. But seek out and find friends who are willing to make positive changes WITH you, and surround yourself with them. And try to be the positive influence on those negative women around you. At some point they may actually change their mindset and join you on your journey! The tribe of women in your life is hugely important in shaping your attitude – so surround yourself with positive women. Get into an accountability group on Facebook or other forum; it does not have to be face-to-face to be effective.

I am not saying I have all the answers. I sure don't have a magic wand or some potion, poultice, or plan that will be an instant fix for your symptoms and you will feel good immediately. It takes a while to find the right combination of natural remedies that work for you, because everyone's body responds differently. What worked well for me may not work so well for you. A little experimentation is sometimes necessary to find the right "fit". Dealing with hormone issues is complicated – it may take a while before you feel like the "old" you again. But one thing I can say for sure: when you follow a healthier, balanced nutrition plan, drink more water, and do moderate exercise, you WILL start to feel the effects of it soon. And the more you do, the more you will feel those positive changes taking place.

You really DO deserve to feel better. But only YOU are in control. Decide that TODAY is THE day that you will take control, make some healthy changes, and start on a journey to better health.

CHANGE YOUR MINDSET: DIET=EDIT

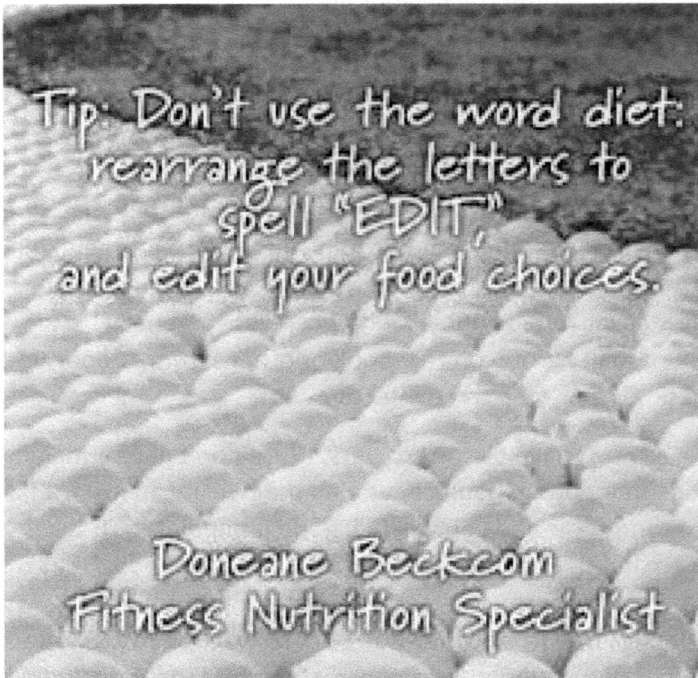

Tip: Don't use the word diet: rearrange the letters to spell "EDIT," and edit your food choices.

Doneane Beckcom
Fitness Nutrition Specialist

One of my favorite things to tell people is to STOP using the word "diet." After all, it IS a four letter word, right? Anyone who has ever been on a diet to lose weight knows that it is not easy, or fun, and often the results are short-lived.

The word diet has a negative connotation. It makes you feel like you have done something wrong and are being punished by having to eat some crazy combination of foods or restrict yourself in a way that is not healthy. Going into a new eating plan with this burden on your mind is just setting yourself up for failure.

I mean, who in her right mind has ever said "I am so excited to be starting a diet on Monday!"

Yep. That's right: NO ONE. EVER!

The problem with so many popular diets that have flooded our newsfeeds in recent years is that they are not balanced – they take away an entire food group, or cut it back so much, or eliminate solid food altogether, that your body ends up with a chemical imbalance which can lead to significant health issues (ketosis, for example, by cutting out carbs; digestive issues from not getting enough "good" bacteria or depleting it by an unhealthy "cleanse;" "brain fog" because your body is lacking healthy carbs, etc.). Once the diet is over, unless you have done something to change your eating habits, all of the old ways of eating and behaving return, along with the weight you lost (and maybe more).

And most people hope – and believe – that they can lose weight fast. On some diets you can, but not in a healthy way, and often not permanently. If it took you three years to gain 30 pounds, it is going to take you a while to take it off. Healthy weight loss that does not tax your body inappropriately is about 1 – 3 pounds per week. More than this and you run the risk of health issues and the likelihood that the weight will not stay off. Slowly losing weight, along with behavior modification, is the BEST way to make a healthy change for the future, resulting in long-term weight loss and better, healthier habits for the rest of your life.

When dieting, people often forget to drink adequate water. Drinking water actually helps you lose weight. You need to drink at least 50% of your body weight in ounces per day. So, if you weigh 120lbs, you should drink 60ozs of water a day. And start the day with a glass of warm water with the juice of one lemon before you drink or eat anything in the morning. This will aid digestion and ramp up your metabolism as well.

You can spice up this recipe, get an energy boost and fight inflammation by using this easy recipe:

- ½ cup filtered water
- Juice of ½ lemon
- 1 tablespoon apple cider vinegar (with "The Mother")
- 1 tablespoon local honey
- 1 teaspoon cinnamon
- ½ teaspoon turmeric
- ¼ teaspoon cayenne pepper

Mix all ingredients in a shaker bottle and drink all at once (this is not a sipping drink!).

Engaging the services of a health coach can mean the difference between developing new healthy habits and reverting to the old habits once the diet is over. Having support and motivation along the way, and AFTER the plan has been executed and you move on to maintenance, are the keys to long-term success with any new habits, whether in nutrition, exercise, daily habits, or whatever else you are trying to change.

Instead of "diet," rearrange the letters to spell "edit," and simply edit your food choices. When you make the decision to eat healthier, you are making the choice to edit what you have been eating. This is a much healthier way to go about making changes in the way you eat, with the goal being habits changed for a lifetime, not just a quick fix to lose weight temporarily. When I work with a client, I never give them a diet to follow, because of the word's negative associations. What I do provide is a plan for eating that meets basic nutritional needs, and meets the client's goals whether it is for weight loss, dealing with menopausal symptoms, building lean muscles, training for a marathon, or just wanting to make healthy lifestyle changes.

My nutrition plans will never leave you hungry or feeling like you are being restricted or deprived.

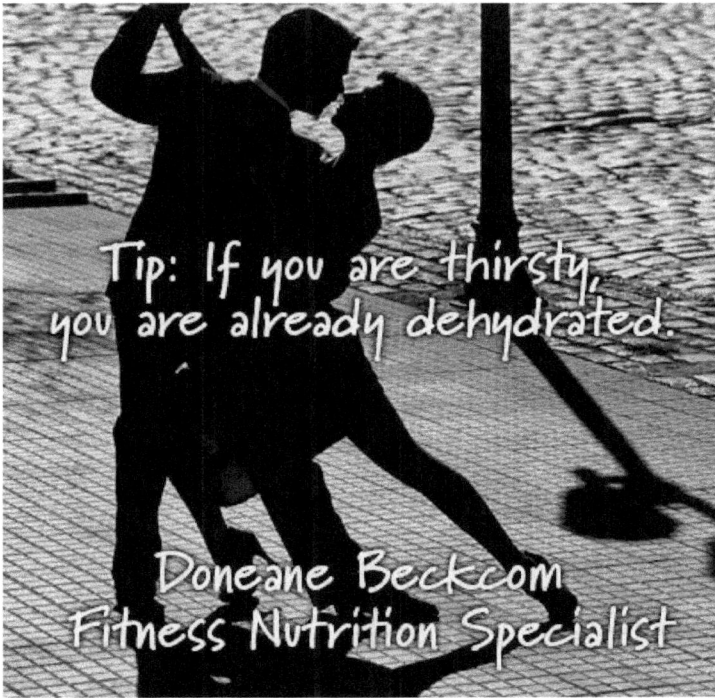

Tip: If you are thirsty, you are already dehydrated.

Doneane Beckcom
Fitness Nutrition Specialist

I encourage you to take the word "diet" out of your vocabulary and mindet and choose to edit your food choices and lifestyle choices instead. This is an easy change. You can make it today.

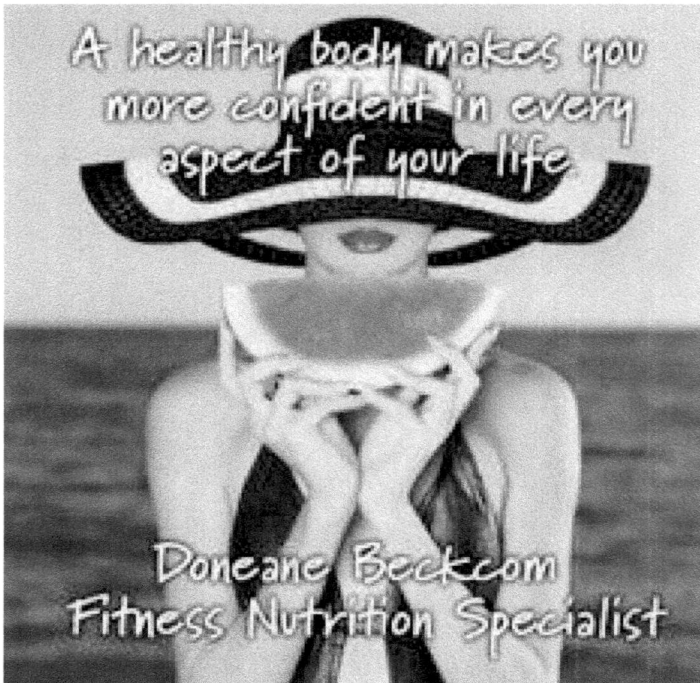

A healthy body makes you more confident in every aspect of your life

Doneane Beckcom
Fitness Nutrition Specialist

I was not always good to my body. I bet you can say that about your body also. When I was in college, I partied all the time, drank WAY too much, had irregular sleep, and ate fast food. Always fast food, always on the go! I still looked good and felt pretty good.

Fast forward to my mid 20s and something happened. All of that hard living started to catch up with me, and I started having health problems. Digestive issues, an ulcer in my esophagus, skin issues, thyroid out of whack – all sorts of stuff. So of course my doctor put me on medication. At that time, I was into fitness and exercise but not so much into nutrition, so taking meds was not a big deal to me – as it is now.

A few years later, after having my daughter, I developed asthma and arthritis. Again, from not taking care of myself and doing the things necessary to keep my insides as healthy as my outsides were looking. I had a horrible bout of pneumonia and was hospitalized for a week and put on more meds. Because I was still not really worried about what I was putting into my body, taking the meds did not bother me.

The stomach meds did not work, the asthma meds made me jittery, and the arthritis meds were taken off the market due to people having heart issues while taking them – and THAT was the ONLY one that worked! OK great, so now I am an asthmatic in constant pain from arthritis and ulcers and I am susceptible to pneumonia. Not a pretty picture.

My physical condition made me feel bad and led me to make really poor decisions in every area of my life. Personal, professional, spiritual, you name it – my life was a mess. By now I was a single mom of a seven-year-old, still popping pills and inhaling potions every day to mask the conditions that made me feel so bad and make dumb decisions.

I finally decided to DO something about how I was feeling. Surely there was something I could do – short of taking all the meds that had nasty side-effects and did not work – that could "fix" my problems. I had always been into exercise, so I decided that I needed to start being good to my insides just like I was being good to my outsides by exercising and staying in shape.

Over the course of about three years, I changed my eating habits and was able to get off of the medications I was taking. And through continued good nutrition choices, I no longer suffer from ulcers, digestive issues, arthritis, or asthma. I do not take ANY medications – none. Zero – and that was about 15 years ago.

Around that time my perimenopausal symptoms started to kick into gear. Thankfully I already knew a few tricks about foods to eat and those to avoid, and supplements to add to my daily intake to combat those symptoms naturally. I did not want to start HRT because of the research that suggested it might be unsafe, or even necessary. Fortunately, my doctor was supportive when I told her that even the low dose birth control she had me on was about to stop.

That is why laying the groundwork for dealing with your symptoms is so important. Even though your body might not be good to you right now, be good to her! The better you take care of your body, the better it will respond to your efforts to live healthier, and the better your chances are of alleviating your symptoms. Be good to your body and she will be good to you!

Now, I am not promising that you can do the same things I have done. But I can tell you that through the years and my own research, trial and MANY errors with nutrition and exercise choices, being my own guinea pig, I became educated in nutrition. You, too, can get on the road to feeling better and dealing with your symptoms. I have helped many people change their eating habits, feel better, control those bothersome symptoms, and bring their lives back into alignment where they experience freedom and joy again. And some were able to get off of medications they had taken for some time.

So, be good to your body, inside and out. Staying healthy is 70% nutrition and 30% exercise. If you get that balance right, you are on the way to better health, a better life, and a better YOU!

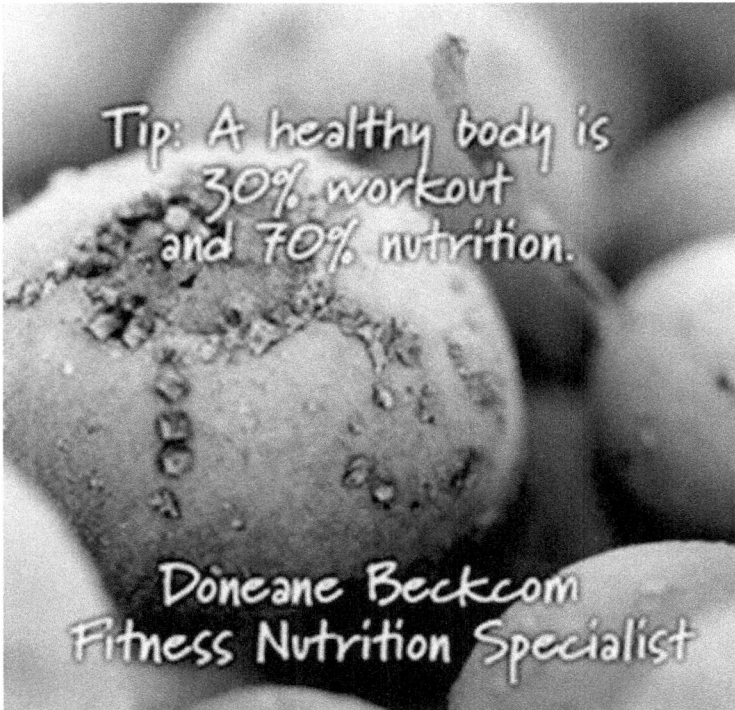

Tip: A healthy body is 30% workout and 70% nutrition.

Doneane Beckcom
Fitness Nutrition Specialist

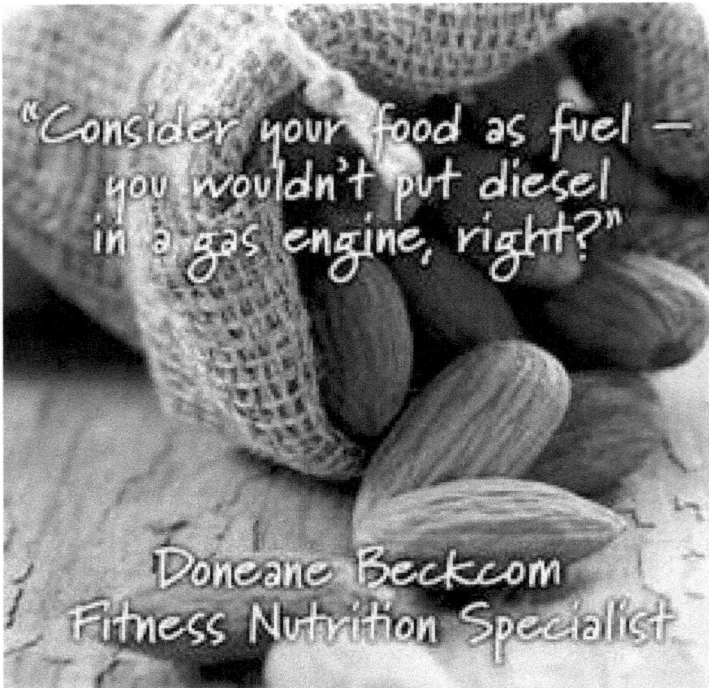

"Consider your food as fuel — you wouldn't put diesel in a gas engine, right?"

Doneane Beckcom
Fitness Nutrition Specialist

You would never put diesel in a gasoline engine, right?

Of course not!

You take good care of your car, don't you? Change the tires, the oil, buy new brake pads, etc. Me too. It's a fine machine and it has to run properly to get me where I need to go. Plus, I LOVE my car!

Isn't your body a fine machine also? Surely you love your body, too (well, you may not love the way it looks all the time, or how it acts right now, but you get my point).

So why do you put chemicals, preservatives, artificial colors and flavors, and other unhealthy things into your body?

IT'S LIKE PUTTING DIESEL IN A GAS ENGINE!

Think about it! You really are putting the wrong things in and expecting to FEEL good! It will NOT happen! In fact, a great deal of what you are eating is probably contributing to the symptoms you may be having right now!

Everything – and I mean EVERYTHING – you eat, drink, rub on, inhale, spray on, soak in, ALL of it is reduced to the microscopic level inside your body. And that affects how everything in your body functions. If you are putting the wrong things in, your body is not going to function and perform to its fullest capability. You will feel sluggish, have brain fog, be unable to concentrate, sleep badly – many of these symptoms boil down to what you are ingesting through your mouth, nose and skin. Because our bodies do not recognize chemicals, artificial ingredients, etc. as food, they spend a lot of energy trying to process and eliminate them as toxins. This heavy chemical load really puts a burden on our bodies.

You don't run your car on empty, do you?

No, of course not! It needs a minimum amount of fuel to function and get you to where you need to be.

Have you ever run out of gas? I have, a few times! It is NOT a fun place to be. So now I always make sure that I refuel BEFORE I need to – before my gas light comes on.

So why don't we treat our bodies the same way? We run on empty ALL the time. Feel hunger pangs in the middle of a 10AM meeting and eat a donut because someone brought donuts just for the meeting. Eat at the wrong time, day or night, eat the wrong things, we have all done this, including me. Totally throwing your blood sugar off balance for the rest of the day, making yourself crave things you should not eat, sure, we 've all done it.

21

But did you know that the really healthy way to eat is NOT to let yourself get hungry? NOT to run on empty. I am sure you have heard the term "hangry," right? Hungry + angry because you are hungry = Hangry. Yep. Been there, ate the wrong things and regretted it later.

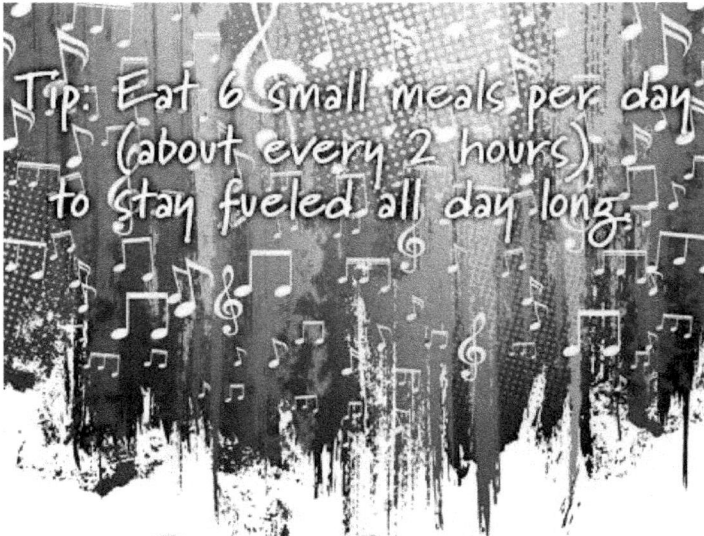

Tip: Eat 6 small meals per day (about every 2 hours) to stay fueled all day long.

Donéane Beckcom
Fitness Nutrition Specialist

Eating six smaller meals per day, one every two to three hours or so, will keep your blood sugar stable during the day, keep you energized and focused, and prevent you from having a "crash" around 3PM because you let yourself get hangry and ate a way-too-big lunch full of carbs! You will be totally amazed at how good you feel once you adjust to this eating schedule.

I know, it sounds strange to anyone who has never done this. But I promise you, it makes total sense and it is easy to accomplish, with a little planning ahead of time. I am talking now about meal prep.

There is not a right or wrong way to meal prep. You have to figure out what works for you, your family, your schedule, and your life. But as an example, here's how I do it:

Saturdays are my meal prep days, and I am out the door at 8AM. I go to the local farmers' market to get the freshest organic local produce and free range organic eggs, then head to the grocery store to get the other things I need for the coming week to prep all of my meals and snacks. To save time, sometimes I place an online grocery order and have it ready to be picked up on my way home. Once I get home and unload, I start chopping, cooking, etc. until everything is done. I have a great stackable steamer that will steam a whole chicken or large fish fillets, cook all of my veggies, and make broth – all at the same time. It is a HUGE time saver. Once everything is cooked, I portion small meals into BPA free reusable containers – breakfast, lunch, and dinner for every day of the week. I even make "salads in a jar" that keep fresh all week in sealed mason jars. I also make enough snacks to have a mid-morning and a mid-afternoon snack while I am at work. Half of the meals go into the freezer to keep for later in the week, and the other half in the fridge that will be eaten within the first couple of days of the week.

And everything you just read is usually done within three to four hours. That may sound like a lot of time in the kitchen, but think about all the time I saved by doing it ALL in one day – this way, meals and snacks can be grabbed as I head out the door, and are ready when I come home for the day. Spending no time in the kitchen after a busy work day? Heck yeah!

I have some great meal prep videos on my YouTube channel and also on my Facebook page and blog. Be sure to check the links at the end of the book for where to go to learn about fueling your body just like you do your car!

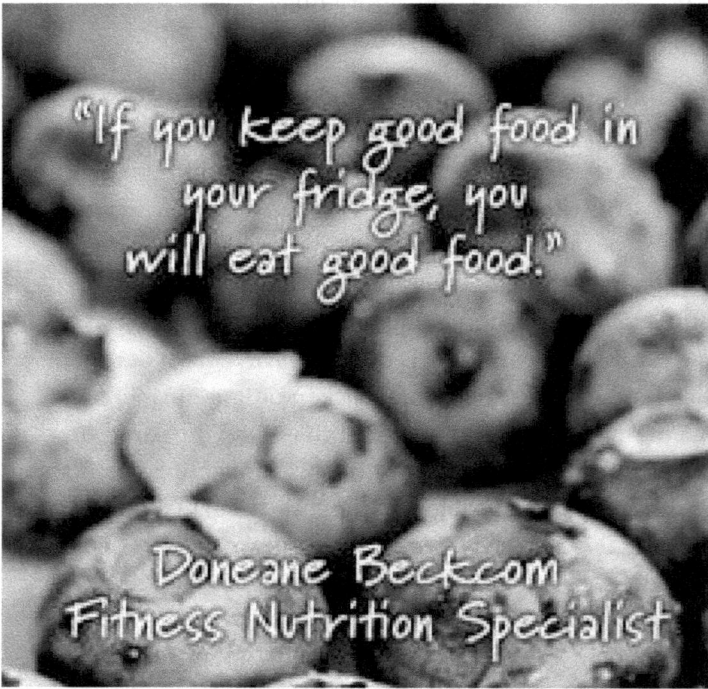

"If you keep good food in your fridge, you will eat good food."

Doneane Beckcom
Fitness Nutrition Specialist

The very first thing I do with a new client is a kitchen clean-out. It is a double lesson, because we also learn about how to read nutrition labels and ingredient lists to determine what is in the product that we may not want to put into our bodies.

The hard part comes when we decide either to toss or keep it, or maybe donate it to a local food pantry or shelter. And what complicates the decision is if you have a spouse or partner in the home, and it's even MORE complicated when you have KIDS! Not everyone will want to join you on your health journey, so you have to adjust. I have lived through that with kids and spouse, so I know it is a struggle.

What I typically do with clients is create a space for "their food" in the pantry and fridge, so that the foods that everyone else in the house is eating are still there, but just not in "your space." Kind of like "out of sight, out of mind" even though it is technically still there. But if you have ZERO willpower when it comes to the cookies, cakes, chips, etc., then you might want to put all of that stuff in bins on the shelf so that you really don't have to see it when you open the pantry or fridge!

When you are ready to clean out your kitchen and fridge, here are a few pointers:

Throw away processed, packaged foods – most contain chemical ingredients, artificial sweeteners, and trans fats. Anything that comes in a bag, box, or can likely contains these things – like high fructose corn syrup, MSG, partially hydrogenated oils, artificial ANYTHING – if you see any of those on the ingredients list, TOSS IT! And be sure to read the entire list of ingredients, as most of the artificial things are at the end (ingredients are listed from the highest quantities to lowest, so the first five on the list are the ones to look at first, but don't stop there!). These ingredients can cause a host of symptoms and aggravate those that already exist in your body, so get rid of them! They cause inflammation and contribute to menopausal symptoms.

Trash old condiments that you hardly use – these are often hidden sources of sugar, sodium and fat, and could harbor mold or bacteria.

Get rid of vegetable or canola oil and replace with organic extra virgin olive oil or coconut oil.

Throw away plastic food containers and purchase BPA-free glass or plastic containers.

Check your non-stick cookware for scratches and rust, and consider replacing them with Teflon-free or ceramic-coated cookware. This option is healthier to cook with and environmentally friendly as well.

Purge your fridge of any "science experiments" hiding in the back or in the crisper bin. I have had a few of those . . . . ☺

So when you get rid of the "bad" stuff that your body does not need, it's time to replace it with the good stuff. This is where learning how to shop healthy comes in. And it takes a while to learn how to do this and get really good at it, so that it does not take you hours in the grocery store. Eating a more natural diet, with lots of fruits and vegetables, will help you to combat the bothersome symptoms you may be experiencing, and will make you healthier overall!

Here are some simple tips to get you started:

When you plan meals, you should automatically take stock of what you have in the pantry and fridge and choose dishes that make use of what you already have. That is rule #1 – effective meal planning and grocery shopping makes use of what is already on hand. And you should always have a bevy of staples at home, to be able to make a healthy meal in a pinch, which I will elaborate on shortly.

As you write down the meals you want to make throughout the week, list the items you need to purchase. This ensures that you have what you need and nothing else. Make sure to include enough foods from each food group, with special attention to fresh vegetables and fruits for every meal as well as snacks. I have several done-for-you meal plans available on my website with the shopping lists already DONE. Check out the links at the end of the book for more info on where to find these great resources, many of which are free!

Tip: Hungry for a snack?
Grab a piece of fruit

Duncane Beckcom
Fitness Nutrition Specialist

At the grocery store, always keep an eye out for sales on whole grain products like brown rice, quinoa pasta, couscous, and steel cut oats so you can stock up and have them as staples to have on hand to make a healthy meal when you may not have a full fridge. Frozen fish, frozen vegetables and even frozen fruit are also good to keep on hand for quick entrées, side dishes and smoothies when you haven't had a chance to buy fresh ingredients. Just do a quick check of the label to be sure that the ONLY added ingredient, if anything, is WATER. Some frozen foods have added sugars, salt, artificial colors and preservatives.

Aside from sale items that are a smart buy, stick to the list on your meal plan and shop the perimeter of the store – this is where the healthier foods are located. Avoiding the inner aisles reduces the likelihood of buying products with little nutritional value – this is where most of the packaged and processed foods are shelved.

Once you make a habit of reading nutrition labels and ingredients lists, you will become more proficient at it and shopping will not take as long. Just be patient, bring a pair of reading glasses if you need them (I think they make the print so small on PURPOSE to discourage us from reading the nutrition labels!) and spend some time reviewing the labels on your favorite products. You will get the hang of it and be healthier for it! Every so often, be sure to re-check the labels on your favorite products, as sometimes the manufacturer makes a change and there could be something in it that you do not want, the amount of sodium has increased, or the serving size and calorie count has changed, etc. Do not rely on reading a label only once – check back often. One of my favorite cereals which had no preservatives in it for YEARS suddenly had a nasty preservative added, and I just happened to check the ingredients list one day and BAM there it was, right at the very end. I was so upset!

Here's a final tip on this topic: not only should you keep good food in the fridge, keep it VISIBLE also. Set out that beautiful crystal bowl that Grandma gave you and fill it with fresh fruit (isn't it just gathering dust in the china hutch?). Keep another bowl or basket on the counter with avocadoes and tomatoes in it. Keep lemons and limes in plain view to cut and squeeze into your water. Keep healthy snacks on your desk at work in plain sight. If you keep good things visible, you will grab those when you want a quick snack.

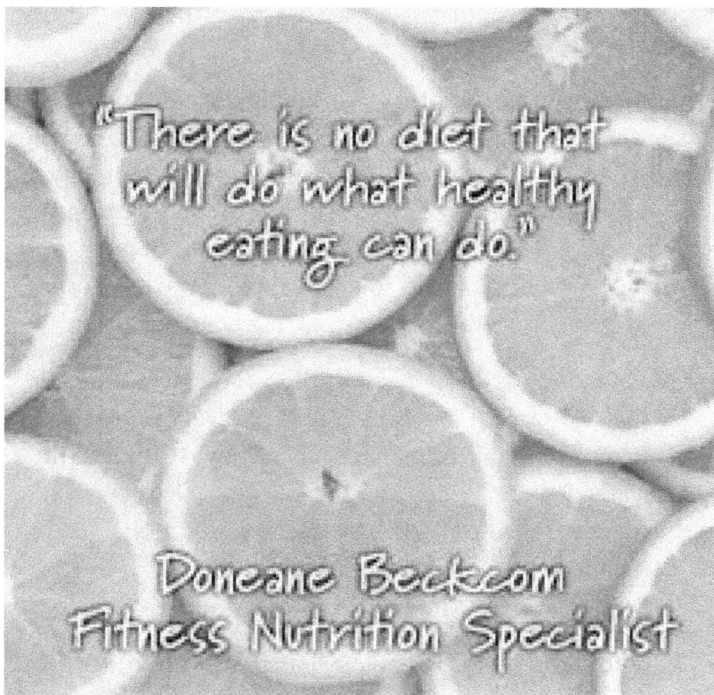

"There is no diet that will do what healthy eating can do."

Doneane Beckcom
Fitness Nutrition Specialist

Earlier in the book I talked about taking the word "diet" out of your vocabulary. I hope that you are seriously considering this! Because there really is not a diet out there that can take the place of simply following a healthy, balanced nutrition plan.

Once you make the choice to edit your food choices and lifestyle habits, you will start to see small noticeable changes in many areas of your life. Remember, Rome wasn't built in a day.

Even so, where you once were "foggy" during the day, you will find more clarity.

Where you were sore and groggy in the morning when getting out of bed, you will wake more rested and refreshed, with less pain in your joints.

Where you lacked energy during the day and felt a "crash" mid-afternoon, you will become more energetic and have fewer ups and downs during the day.

All of these changes can be attributed to making very small changes in the way you eat: cutting out "bad" carbs and eating whole grains instead, cutting out foods that cause inflammation and substituting those that combat it, drinking plenty of water, and eating more frequent (and healthier) meals during the day to control blood sugar dips and spikes. Simple, small, easily attainable steps which will help you improve your health.

These simple changes are the best way to move toward better habits for the rest of your life. Trying to do an "all or nothing" approach to making healthy changes will not work. It takes at least 21 days to change a habit, so making small changes over the course of several weeks is the best way to see a change and have it "stick."

Think about it – most likely, you have been living the same way and eating the same things for many years at this point. Or, you slipped into some not-so-healthy habits a few years ago and just cannot get back to where you know you should be. And that is ok! For as long as it took you to get into the bad habits, it is going to take you a while to reverse and replace them with healthier ones. Give yourself time. Do not get discouraged. That is why it is important to be in an accountability group, such as my Facebook group. When you are ready to get started, I would love to have you join us. The link to join the group is in the resources at the end of the book.

There are no fad diets or quick fixes that can replace what healthy eating can do for your body. Remember when I said that everything you eat and drink affects your body down to the microscopic level? It is true! When you start replacing the unhealthy things you eat and drink with healthier things, your cells become healthier, which can slow down the aging process, slow down or halt disease processes altogether, alleviate bothersome symptoms, and make you feel better!

I am living proof that this works! I had terrible eating habits (and some other bad health habits) and my health really was poor. Once I changed my habits, I started to feel better. I was amazed at how bad I had been feeling before! I never want to feel that way again. I want you to be able to say that someday!

Two old phrases come to mind here: Nancy Reagan's drug prevention slogan, "Just Say No," and Nike's popular ad campaign, "Just Do It." You have to have the mindset to say "No" to anything that is not healthy – food, beverages, activities – and to just "do" those things that are good for you and will lead to better habits and a healthier lifestyle. It really is up to you!

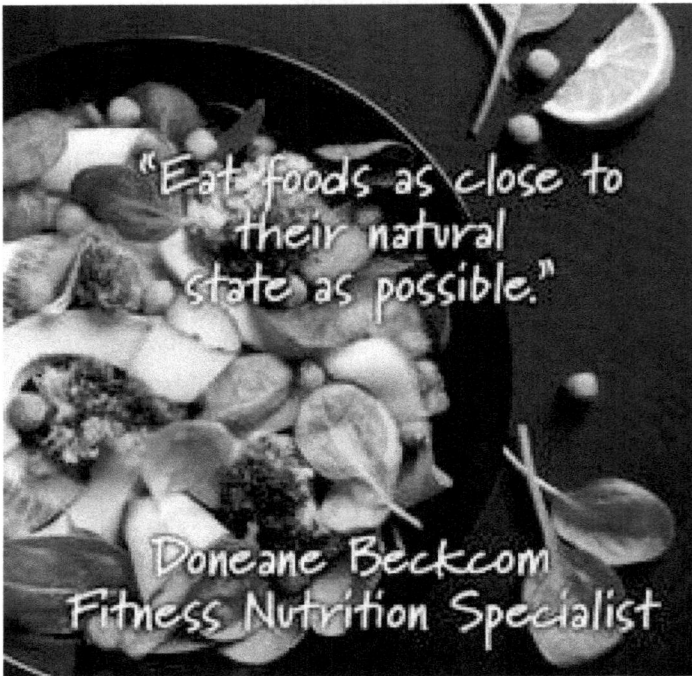

"Eat foods as close to their natural state as possible."

Doneane Beckcom
Fitness Nutrition Specialist

Eat foods as close to their natural state as possible. A daily intake of natural fruits and vegetables, together with lean proteins and healthy fats, is the best way to eat.

What do I mean by foods that are in their "natural state"?

A great example of this idea that you can find in every grocery store is potatoes. Potatoes come in all types: from real ones in the produce department to instant dehydrated potato flakes, potato chips, frozen French fries, shoestring potatoes, potato gnocchi, frozen mashed potatoes, the list goes on and on.

But the best are the REAL ones in the produce department. Yes, they are inconvenient, as they must be washed, peeled, sliced, cooked, mashed, etc. But think of what you are saving your body from by eating a real potato as opposed to a processed version: added chemicals, flavors, emulsifiers, colors, etc.

This idea can be applied to EVERY food. Real mixed fruit or fruit-in-a-cup with added sugar syrup? Real asparagus or frozen asparagus (with artificial ingredients) to pop in the microwave? Real whole grain breads or "wheat" bread colored with molasses and containing high fructose corn syrup? Real, range free, grain fed lean beef or beef from antibiotic-laden-hormone-infused-inhumanely-treated cattle?

The list is endless, like the aisles in the grocery stores crowded with shoppers who are wasting their time, health and money. (Sorry, I get "aisle rage" in the grocery store, seeing all the people shopping without a clue).

But I digress ...

This brings back into play the idea of healthy shopping. Think about your favorite grocery store right now, in your mind's eye. Aren't all the healthy items on the perimeter of the store? Fruits and vegetables, meats, poultry, the fish market, dairy, all of them are around the outside aisles of the store. There are exceptions, with healthy frozen foods, gluten free, "health" foods that might be on an inner aisle. But for the most part, if you shop in a "traditional" grocery store, this is the set up. The inner aisles have all of the processed junk, chips, cookies, cake mixes, prepackaged dinners, things meant to have a "shelf life." Again, there are exceptions and sometimes there are a few healthy items in these inner aisles, but the majority of unhealthy products are located here. Foods that are meant to sit on a shelf in a package, by and large, contain unhealthy ingredients meant to preserve and extend their shelf life – things like high fructose corn syrup and trans fats (hydrogenated oils). A product meant to sit on the shelf in your pantry is likely to contain these unnatural substances, which are downright unhealthy.

Research shows that foods not in their natural state, containing added artificial ingredients, contribute to menopausal symptoms, inflammatory diseases such as arthritis and asthma, and digestive issues. When you cut out these foods and replace them with real natural food, your body will start to detox from all of the garbage it has been fed, and you WILL begin to feel better!

Why consume all of that unnatural garbage when you can spend just a little more time preparing your foods from the real versions and not the 'Franken food' processed ones? I would rather take the extra time, knowing that I am not putting something artificial into my body. Yes, it's less convenient and sometimes more expensive, but if you want to get healthy and feel better from the inside out, this is a necessary choice, one that you MUST make.

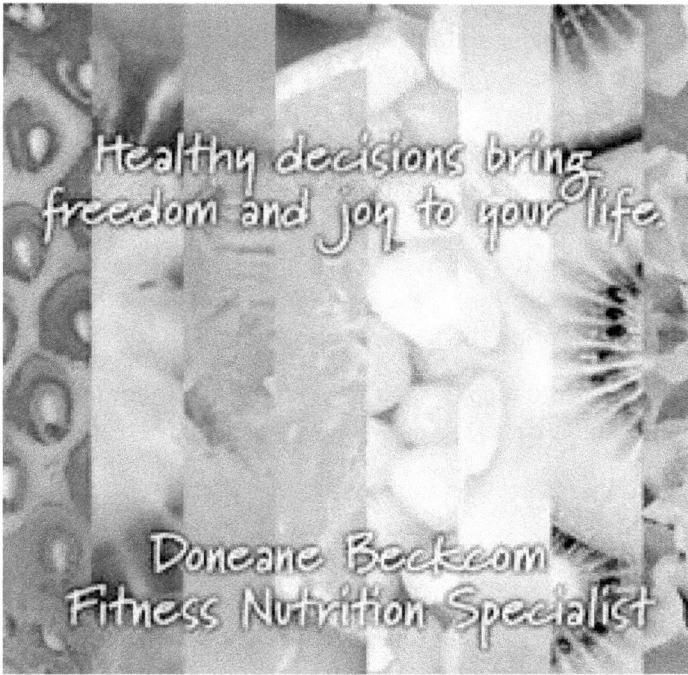

Healthy decisions bring freedom and joy to your life.

Doneane Beckcom
Fitness Nutrition Specialist

When you start to make healthier decisions, you will begin to see changes in other areas of your life as well. Feeling better and getting rid of bothersome symptoms is one thing, but having the freedom to really enjoy is something else!

I will give you a real life example from my own journey.

Earlier I talked about my health issues that caused me to make some serious life changes. I was taking several different medications multiple times per day. So I had to build time into my life to be able to take them. Swallowing a bunch of pills and liquids and inhaling three different types of asthma medication was time consuming – to say nothing of the unpleasant side-effects.

Cut to when I decided to take charge of my health starting with my nutrition. Once I began to make healthier decisions, the freedom of NOT having to take all of the medications, which I had been taking for so many years, was liberating. No longer did I have to get up earlier to start the medical merry-go-round. No longer did I have to excuse myself from lunch with co-workers or dinner with friends to go into the bathroom to take some medication that I did not want to gulp in front of people. No more monthly trips to the pharmacy or check-ups at the doctor just to get my prescriptions renewed for yet another six-month supply. Not to mention the money I was saving!

I had a level of joy in my life again that I had not experienced in a long time. And most of it was because I just FELT better!

Feeling better physically is important to every aspect of our daily lives. If you feel bad when you get out of bed, chances are you are not going to spend a lot of time getting ready for your day. Not spending time fixing your hair just right, or picking out that perfect suit or outfit for the day's work or events. Or maybe while you are at work and still not feeling good, an important decision needs to be made. If you are not in the right frame of mind because you do not feel good physically, all of your decisions are going to be stilted toward the You that does not feel 100% all the time.

I know. I have been there and made those not-so-healthy decisions. And healthy decisions are not just about your health, or your nutritional plan, or your exercise routine. You can make unhealthy decisions in EVERY area of your life – work, relationships, activities you participate in – all of these decisions can be 'healthy' or 'unhealthy' depending upon your mindset. So part of the journey toward feeling better physically is also making sure that emotionally, spiritually, psychologically, you are bringing those parts of yourself along for the ride.

Getting your symptoms under control, weaning off medications, learning a healthier way of eating, beginning to engage in moderate exercise, whatever you need to do to start feeling better and making healthier decisions – will you make the decision to get started today?

I have given you some ideas in the previous chapters and laid the groundwork for choices you need to consider. So now let's dive into some things you can do, and things you should NOT do, in order to overcome your symptoms. Research I conducted before writing this book revealed that the number one symptom that was disrupting women's lives was hot flashes, closely followed by night sweats and insomnia. Weight gain and bladder control issues followed as the bottom two. The big top three symptoms we are going to tackle in the coming chapters. If you get those under control, the others will often lessen as well.

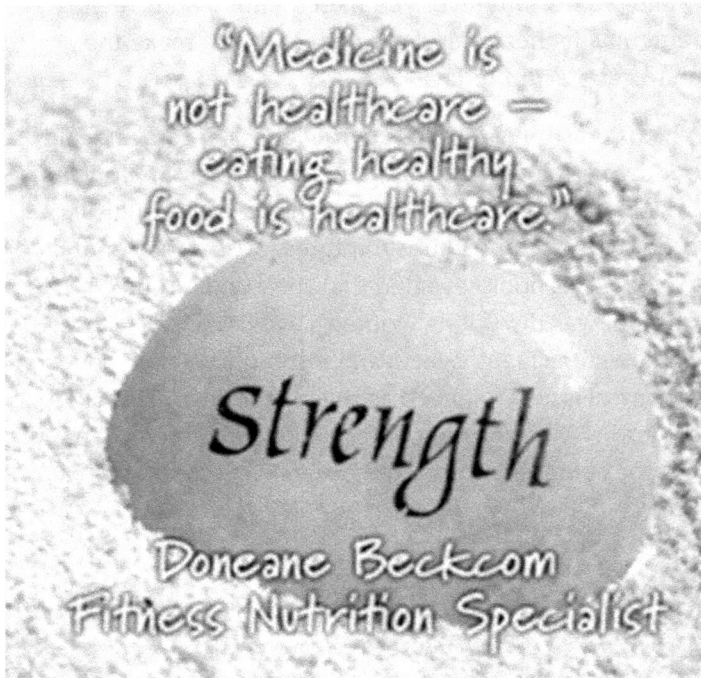

"Medicine is not healthcare — eating healthy food is healthcare"

Strength

Doneane Beckcom
Fitness Nutrition Specialist

So many people tell me, when I begin to design a new nutrition plan for them, that it is "too time consuming" or "too hard because I have kids" or "I don't have time because of work/spouse/kids/whatever." Or, feeling cruddy has become so commonplace that you think nothing will change it.

Sister, there is always room for change and improvement. Always!

The bottom line is, only you can determine when you are ready to make healthy changes in your life. I cannot tell you when that time is, only you can make that choice. It took me a lot of years of not feeling well, dealing with symptoms, and making poor choices to do something about it – finally! You may not be at that point yet, and that's okay. To make a choice and stick to it, you really have to WANT it for you. You cannot do it because someone else wants you to, or because your doctor wants you to, or because you are trying to please someone other than yourself. Only then will the changes take place and actually last over the course of your lifetime. You have to be at the point of being ready and willing to make that change.

Face it, bad food choices are an addiction. I know because I was there: addicted to sugar, fried foods, fast foods, all the things that were bad for me. And someone who is addicted to something cannot, and will not, make a change until he or she is ready for it. No "intervention" will work unless the addict is at the point of making a change for themselves. I know this, because my husband is my worst nutrition client! I harped on him for years to change his eating habits, but it wasn't until his doctor told him (for about the fifth time) that he was borderline Type 2 diabetic, and put him on two medications, that he changed his habits. No amount of love, cajoling, begging, screaming made a difference to him. The choice had to be his when he was ready.

And when you do get to that point, you can and will find the strength to do what is necessary to get healthy again, to feel better again. It may not come from your family and friends, you may have to find support in a totally different place, and Facebook Groups are a great place to start when you are beginning a new journey when it comes to making healthy changes.

When you are ready, I will be honored to have you join my group! We keep each other accountable, share our successes and failures, post healthy recipes and motivational topics, plus it is a great place to garner support, friendship, accountability, and motivation to stay the course.

One of the first things I have a new nutrition client do is assess their daily water intake (we touched on this topic early on but I did not elaborate). Most people do not drink enough water and stay in a constant state of partial dehydration. This can exacerbate hormonal symptoms BIG time. You should be drinking at least half of your body weight in ounces per day. So if you weigh 140 pounds, you should drink 70 ounces of water per day. Most folks cringe and say "That's too much; no way can I drink that much water." Well, the truth is, YES you can! And once you get used to it, your body will crave it, and it will become a new healthy habit. Our bodies are about 85% water anyway; even our bones have water in them. Your brain is also high in water content, so when you don't drink enough, you are depriving your body of an essential part of its very existence! If one of your symptoms is brain fog, chances are that along with the hormonal imbalance, you are partially dehydrated all the time. Increasing your water consumption can also aid in weight loss, if that is your goal.

Drinking more water has the added benefit of detoxifying your system and flushing out those things that you have been putting in that are not so healthy. Your liver, kidneys, and digestive track will become healthier with more water intake, since they function better with adequate water intake. Your skin will also become healthier. Muscles will become more flexible; your skin will glow again. The benefits to your body are really amazing by just upping your daily water intake.

If drinking more water (and less sodas, tea, and coffee) is the ONLY healthy change you can make right now, GO FOR IT! You have to start somewhere. Just give up one can of soda per day and replace it with a glass of water. Work your way up to drinking the recommended amount of water per day. And play around with it – experiment with infusion bottles, put fruit and herbs in your water (there are some great recipes for this on my

YouTube channel, check out the links at the end of the book), experiment with different flavor enhancers (fruits and herbs, lemon zest or orange zest) and find something that satisfies you so that the experience of shifting to more water is pleasant and does not seem like a chore.

Find a reusable water bottle, BPA free plastic or stainless steel, and take note of how many ounces it holds when full. Calculate your daily intake, and then figure out how many of those bottles you must drink to meet your goal. Believe me, it makes it a less daunting task when you do it this way.

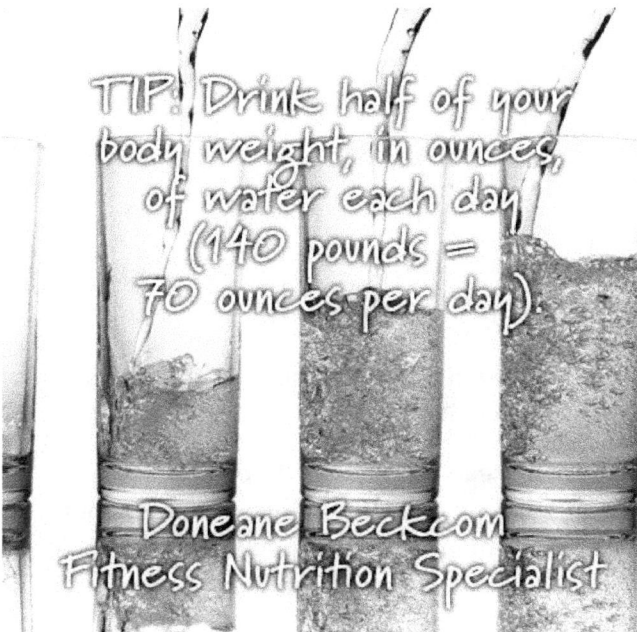

TIP! Drink half of your body weight, in ounces, of water each day (140 pounds = 70 ounces per day).

Doneane Beck.com
Fitness Nutrition Specialist

You DO have the strength to make a change! Baby steps, sister! You CAN do it!

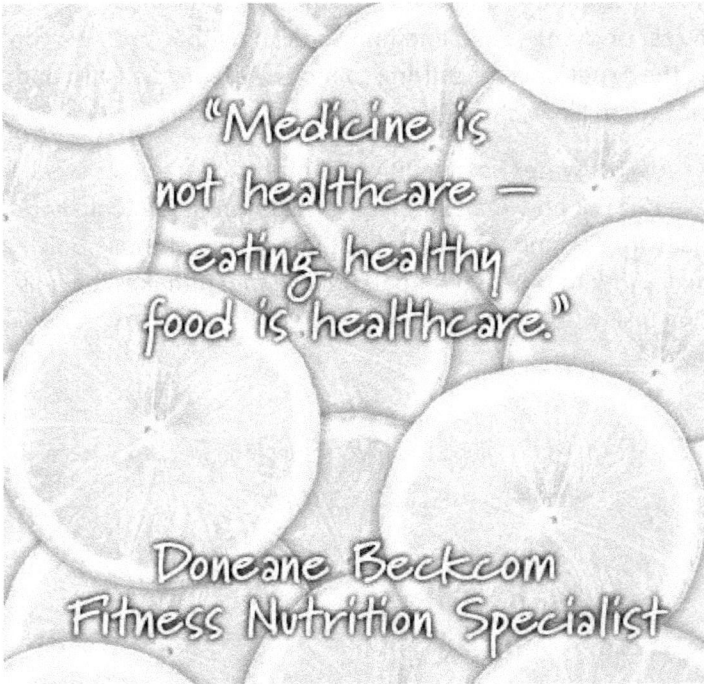

"Medicine is not healthcare — eating healthy food is healthcare."

Doneane Beckcom
Fitness Nutrition Specialist

I think you would agree with this statement: The United States medical system is broken. Right?

Doctors are driven by health insurance companies, which are driven by federal agencies, and we don't want to talk about what drives our government. Requiring people to have health insurance and then punishing them when they don't is just a broken, messed up system. Why can't doctors just do their jobs and keep us healthy instead of needing permission to treat certain conditions in a certain way?

In reality, medicine is NOT healthcare. It certainly isn't preventative healthcare. Eating a balanced blend of healthy foods should be the primary source of everyone's healthcare. If you eat "clean," chances are you will suffer less from diseases, and symptoms you may be experiencing will start to subside. The healthier you keep your insides, the stronger your immune system will be to fight everyday things that can drag you down and make you feel bad – and be ready to fight something more serious like the flu or a staph infection.

You have already read about how I changed my eating habits and got off of the medications I was taking for a variety of health issues. So many things we suffer from are due to what we do or do not eat. Foods that cause inflammation are probably the number one cause of disease. Eating inflammatory foods can also greatly enhance the symptoms of peri- and post-menopause. Sugar is addictive and it's in most processed food. Sodium is bad for you in large amounts and it, too, is in many manufactured foods. When you make the decision to really scrutinize what you eat, you will be surprised at the chemical load you are forcing your body to process.

Add to that load the medications you are taking. A friend and colleague once told me "You cannot poison yourself back to good health." Meaning, that medicine is poison, and rather than taking medicine/poison why not get to the root cause of the problem – which is often poor nutrition. There is also the belief that all disease originates in our digestive system, which makes sense because that is where your immune system "lives." If your gut is not healthy because of wrong foods and poisoning it with medication, then of course your immune system will not be as strong and you will not be able to fight off even simple things like a cold, or something more serious.

And what about all of this "disease resistant" bacteria and infections we keep hearing about? They are caused, in part, by over-prescribing medications, particularly antibiotics, or the patient not taking them correctly, which can cause the bacteria to become resistant, creating "super bugs." Gone are the days of getting a simple shot of a mild antibiotic – now doctors are getting out the "big guns" of medicines that you could get only via IV in the ICU just a few years ago, and giving this to people for a simple sore throat. Doctors have finally figured out that giving children with ear infections an antibiotic is not the best treatment, or even an effective treatment, as many ear issues are viral, not bacterial, and should be allowed run their course, with something to control the ear pain only.

Because of our broken healthcare system and the fact that insurance companies are driving what doctors are able to do, the simple, common-sense solution of eating healthy has gone out the window.

WE NEED TO CHANGE THIS!

If you are taking medications, why not discuss with your doctor if there is an alternative. Can you wean yourself off medications by losing weight, eating better, exercising? To combat diseases and symptoms you are taking meds for, should you consider eating an anti-inflammatory diet or an alkaline diet? These are all smart questions to ask your doctor, if you are ready to make this change in your life. If you are on HRT and want to stop, why not talk to your doctor about natural alternatives?

PLEASE – I am NOT suggesting that you stop taking medications prescribed by your doctor. Depending upon your health history, that could be dangerous. What I am suggesting is that you explore options other than taking a handful of pills every day, or taking shots of something, or inhaling something else. You will not know unless you ask, and do some research on your own so that you are informed about what your doctor advises.

So, what are some of the natural options to control the top three bothersome menopause symptoms?

First, drink plenty of water and get off of processed foods with added sugars. Eating foods closer to their natural source, more fruits and vegetables, and more water will be a great place to start.

Second, start doing moderate exercise. Yoga (my personal favorite), swimming, bike riding, walking, group classes, anything to get you moving and off of the couch! You do NOT have to join a gym. Local churches in your area may have yoga or other fitness classes for a small drop-in fee. I know in my area there are many options available besides joining a gym. So NO excuses!!

Third, consider some natural supplements to combat symptoms. The biggest symptom that disrupts my life is insomnia. I LOVE my sleep! For a long time, I couldn't remember the last time I slept through the night without having to get up to use the bathroom, or just wake up for no reason and not go back to sleep. So here is my remedy (and it is all natural):

- Eat your last meal 2+ hours before bedtime, and make it the smallest, lightest meal of the day. A green salad with 4 ounces of grilled chicken or salmon is plenty for an evening meal, along with a glass of water.
- Have a bedtime routine that is the same every night. My Fitbit alerts me at 8:30PM that it is "time to wind down and get some rest." My goal is to be in bed by 9PM. This is SO important, because it tells your body that it is time to unwind and go to sleep. Disruption to this pattern can cause your body to get off kilter and not transition into sleep mode.
- Do some moderate exercise to rev up your resting metabolism and also relax you for sleep. Yoga is my exercise of choice. About 15 minutes of stretching, breathing, and meditation is all I need. Don't do anything that is cardio in nature. You do not want to raise your heartrate before bed

- Have a protein snack about 30 minutes before bed. Nothing heavy, just a scoop of protein powder in six ounces of non-dairy milk (cashew milk is my favorite)
- Take a warm bath with one cup of Epsom salts (magnesium sulfate which aids in sleep), one cup baking soda (draws out toxins) and a few drops of lavender essential oil (aids in sleep)
- Consider taking a few supplements to help with your symptoms (check with your doctor first!)

> Supplements to aid in sleep (these are suggested amounts; PLEASE consult your doctor first!):
>
> - 250 mg magnesium (less if you also take an Epsom salt bath)
> - 500 – 1000 mg calcium (talk to your doctor about dosing for your age/stage in menopause)
> - 1000 – 2000 IU Vitamin D3 (ditto the above)
> - 100 mg L-Theanine
> - 500 mg L-Tryptophan
> - 3 – 5 mg Melatonin (adjust if you feel groggy the next day)
> - 50 mg zinc
>
> Supplements to take to help with other nighttime symptoms that may interrupt sleep (hot flashes, night sweats)
>
> - 500 mg Turmeric (fights inflammation)
> - Probiotic with 15 - 30 Billion Live Active Cultures
> - 500 mg Evening Primrose Oil
> - 20 – 80 mg Black Cohosh (less if your symptoms are less severe)

Some of these will come in a combined tablet, such as one tablet containing magnesium, calcium, zinc, and D3. The others, which are amino acids that can promote sleep, can be found in a combined tablet (along with zinc and magnesium) known as "ZMA" on the market (stands for zinc, magnesium, and amino acids). I tried ZMA and found that the levels of each ingredient were a little too high for me (I woke up groggy and had diarrhea – NOT how I want to start the day!) I decided to get the separate ingredients so that I could manipulate the dosage amounts until I found what worked for me.

Which brings me back to the point that what works for me may not work for you. Our bodies all react differently to supplements, so you need to be your own research subject (once you have your doctor's approval) to find the dosage amount and timing that works for you.

Take caution with "proprietary blends" of herbs that are sold under various names. Many of these also contain soy, which most doctors will tell us to limit our intake of as we get older, especially if you are already in menopause. If you must have soy, consider eating only fermented types (tofu or edamame). And most of these blended supplements contain other ingredients that you do not need, like artificial colors, flavors, fillers, etc. Check the labels on ALL of the supplements you purchase to be sure that you are not getting anything artificial.

Other supplements that are recommended by non-HRT proponents are Vitamins A, B (all of them!), C, D, E, along with antioxidants such as CoQ-10 and Resveratrol, and essential minerals. You should discuss dosage with your physician, as your age, weight, and other medications can have a bearing on what is recommended for you.

And, ask your doctor about "bio-identical" hormones. This is a non-HRT therapy that uses real hormones derived from plants, as opposed to synthetic ones (from animals) that are chemically altered and are NOT identical to our own hormones. Bio-identical hormones are recognized by our bodies as the same hormones our bodies used to produce when we were younger, before the "change" started to occur. Getting the correct hormones and the proper dosage is for you and your doctor to decide, AFTER appropriate hormone testing. Depending upon your particular symptoms, you may need progesterone and another woman estrogen, or you may need more testosterone (yes, women have it, too!) while another woman needs less. Your doctor can prescribe bio-identical hormones, which are made in compounding pharmacies. Some are even available over the counter, but unless you have been tested and KNOW exactly what you need and what dosage, doing this on your own can be tricky (like taking too much of one hormone and all of a sudden you have facial and chest hair!). But I caution you to do your research, talk to your doctor, talk to a naturopath or compounding pharmacist in your area, get tested, and see if it is right for you. It is one alternative to traditional HRT and is safer, according to studies and research, as far as side-effects and the potential for diseases related to HRT and non-HRT therapies.

Again, I cannot stress enough that you need to discuss adding supplements or other non-HRT therapies to your daily intake with your doctor, especially if you are on other prescription medications or suffer from chronic health issues. Some doctors are willing to let you try natural remedies and will be supportive; others will poo-poo the idea. Find a naturopath in your area and visit with him or her if your own doctor will not be cooperative.

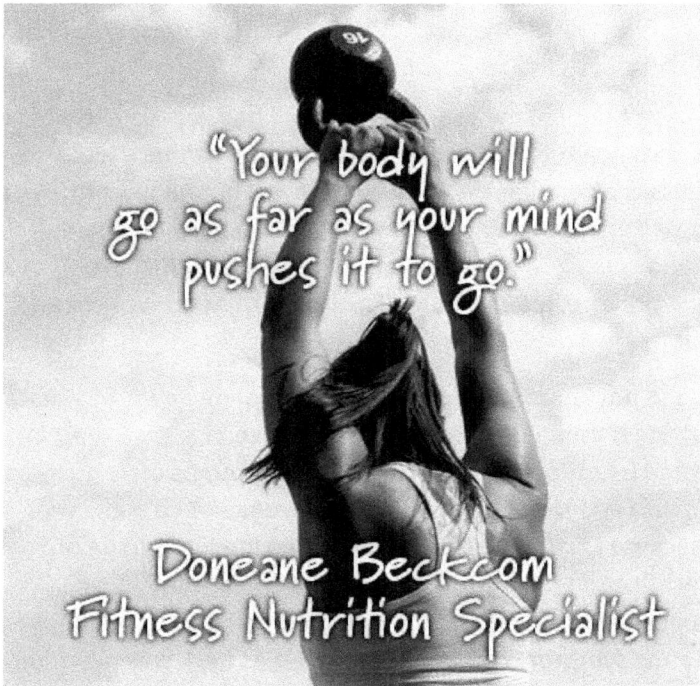

"Your body will go as far as your mind pushes it to go."

Doneane Beckcom
Fitness Nutrition Specialist

I started doing yoga when I was in my 20s, long before it was popular in Texas where I lived at the time. I am sure people in California were already doing it, but in all of the local gyms where I worked or exercised when I was not working, there were no yoga instructors. I was teaching aerobics and weight training, but the grace, flow, and peace of yoga really appealed to me.

So I bought some books and a video tape and learned it at home. Aerobics was a big deal (as were those silly fitness contests which are now all over YouTube and hysterical to watch all these years later!), so I got a certification and started teaching aerobic classes in the local gyms. No one was interested in yoga, even though I offered to get certified to instruct.

I was on my own.

But it wasn't until many years later, after I had moved away for a time and then returned to my hometown, that there were any yoga classes offered at the local gyms. I was not happy with them, so I kept doing it on my own, and then finally found a friend and colleague who was certified, did a great job at teaching practice, and so I joined a class with other women and had some fun.

What I did not know while I was practicing on my own was that I was setting myself up for the one type of exercise that, later in life, would be my saving grace from the symptoms of menopause and the other health issues I developed along the way. Because I found Yoga so helpful, I decided to pursue my own certification in Hatha Yoga, and also in Yoga for Menopause. If it could help me with the awful and sometimes debilitating symptoms I was having, I sure as heck wanted other women to know ALL about it!

Yoga is all about the mind/body connection, and the larger connection between the body/universe. More than any other form of exercise, yoga requires you to focus on your breathing and your body movements from feet to head, and to experience the energy that the body actively or passively releases during each pose. It is a peaceful, relaxing, yet invigorating work out. The ladies who are in my classes are always astonished that the slow, graceful, and purposeful movements we do in an hour long class will make them sweat profusely, shake uncontrollably with muscle fatigue, increase their heart rate, and feel sore the next day (after getting the best night sleep EVER!).

There are many very easy yoga poses that aid in combatting the symptoms of menopause. Exercises that strengthen the pelvic floor muscles to assist in bladder leakage control, strengthen the back and abdominal muscles to deal with cramps and muscle ache that can come with irregular periods and heavy flow, that help the bones to stay strong and less likely to fracture as we age, that reduce stress and promote restful sleep, and that stimulate nerves in the body that can lessen hot flashes and night sweats. I know, it sounds impossible, right? With regular practice, yoga can be the catalyst that turns your symptom-filled days and nights into productive and restful ones. When I began my certification in yoga for menopause and practiced the "new" moves and muscle contractions I was learning, I was amazed when my next cycle came. I usually would have tell-tale signs for a few days: horrible backache (like back labor, if you ever had that in child birth), terrible cramps, moodiness, bloating, brain fog, and then a very heavy flow for about a week. None of that happened! No symptoms (in fact, my period started and I did not even know!) and my flow was much lighter and lasted for fewer days. And it was after just a few weeks of training in this new way that I had this huge change in my symptoms. They have been better ever since!

And yoga is not hard! Yes, some of the more advanced poses take years of practice to perfect (if you follow me on Facebook and saw the "Crow Pose" challenge during the summer of 2016, that's one of them), but anyone can do beginner yoga, from children to elderly people. There is a yoga method and easy poses that literally everyone can do. It does not take any special skill or technique, just a well-trained, dedicated, and compassionate Yogi who will gently guide and direct you as you learn. Just as a baby has to crawl before it can walk, Yogis understand this and do not force a new student to do anything outside their realm of comfort and ability. It is a compassionate, gentle, loving, and peaceful environment in a Yoga class with a well-trained Yogi instructing.

Yoga should never hurt. Even though some of the poses look painful, they should not be. The poses are intended to be gentle, help you to become more flexible, focus on your breathing and the energy force behind the pose. Many Yogis will develop classes that speak to different groups of people – menopausal women, men with low testosterone, pregnant women, kids with ADD/ADHD, people with arthritis – the list is endless that Yoga can help lessen or alleviate altogether.

My personal experience with Yoga, together with eating healthier, allowed me to stop taking medication for arthritis. Yes, I still have it, but the pain and stiffness I experienced every morning and which persisted throughout the day is no longer as pronounced as it was. The same is true with asthma. No more meds, no more asthma attacks, and all from continued healthy eating and Yoga practice. Menopausal symptoms – some are gone and others are much reduced. I am confident that with continued practice throughout my journey into actual menopause, my symptoms are going to improve even more.

I bet yours will too, if you will give it a try! There are some resources at the end of the book for Yoga practice that I hope you will take advantage of.

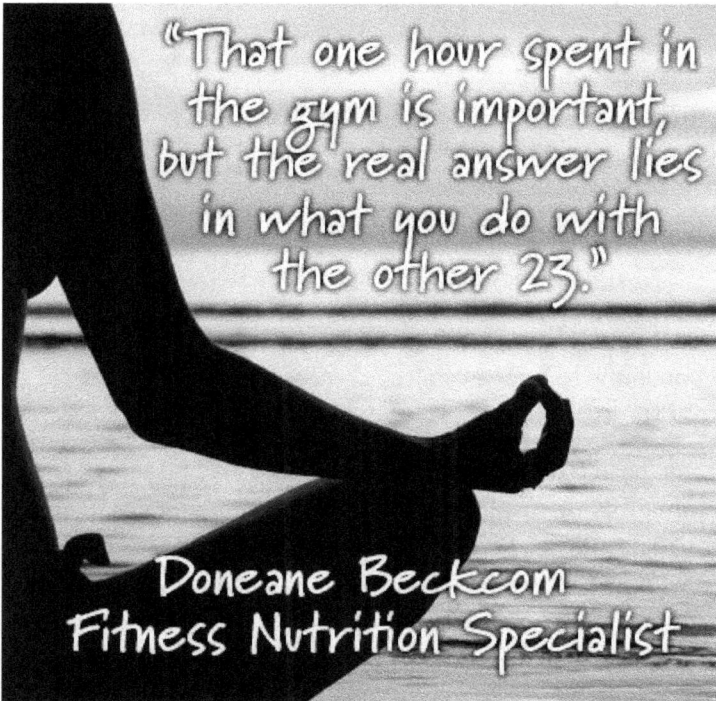

"That one hour spent in the gym is important, but the real answer lies in what you do with the other 23."

Doneane Beckcom
Fitness Nutrition Specialist

All day, every day, we make choices. These choices can be good or bad, healthy or unhealthy, move us forward or set us back. The beauty of it is, the choice you make is all your own.

What is the first choice of the day? For me, it's whether to snooze one more time. Seriously, I am NOT a morning person. Try as I might to get up early and accomplish things does not work for me. Yes, I do get up early, but I have to ease into wakefulness. I am not bounding out of bed and into my Yoga practice immediately. Give me a round of coffee and let me sit with my back on my heating cushion for a few minutes, pet my dogs – only then I can start to feel human.

But what other choices do you make during the day? Choices that influence your psyche, those that have a lasting effect on you or others, are you at your best when you make these decisions? Do you eat that donut or skip it for your protein bar instead? Do you agree to go to lunch with co-workers only to find there is nothing suitable on the menu and you go off plan again? Do you make plans to go to the gym and then let something get in the way?

I get it, sister! I have done ALL of that many times.

Be intentional. Be in control. Do not let others get in the way of what you know to be the healthy choices you need to make, whether they are about what to eat, when to exercise, or important business decisions.

To combat menopausal symptoms, the best thing you can do is to choose natural and anti-inflammatory foods. Processed foods, with all the unnatural additives, can cause inflammation. Here is another list of foods that can contribute to inflammation and menopausal symptoms:

- Sugar (in sodas, candies, cookies, cakes)
- Vegetable oils
- Refined flour
- Fried foods
- Processed meats
- Prepackaged meals
- Dairy
- Artificial sweeteners
- Artificial additives (preservatives, colors, emulsifiers)

Here are some foods that you can add to your daily intake that fight the inflammatory process:

- Organic tomatoes
- Olive oil

- Green leafy vegetables, such as spinach, kale, and collards (look for organic varieties
- Nuts such as almonds and walnuts
- Fatty fish – salmon, mackerel, tuna, and sardines (wild caught is best)
- Fruits such as strawberries, blueberries, cherries, and oranges (organic, especially for the berries)

In addition, eating foods that are more alkaline than acidic can also help your body become healthier, strengthen your immune system, and aid in dealing with bothersome symptoms. Here is just a small list:

VEGETABLES	SPICES AND SEASONINGS
Beets	All herbs
Cruciferous veggies	Chili pepper
Greens and other green veggies	Cinnamon
Orange veggies	Curry
Peppers	Ginger
Radishes	Mustard
	Sea salt
FRUITS	OTHER
Apple	Alkaline water
Apricot	Apple cider vinegar
Banana	Duck and quail eggs
Berries	Mineral water
Orange fruits	Sour dairy products
Watermelon	Veggie juices
NUTS	SUPPLEMENTS
Almonds	Calcium
Chestnuts	Magnesium
	Potassium
	Sodium

Did you notice that there are no animal proteins on that list? This is because all animal protein is acidic, even the "good for you" protein. So, everything in moderation. Your intake should be about 75% alkaline and 25% acidic, if you eat animal proteins at all.

Other things you need to add to your nutrition plan to combat symptoms and improve overall health are things like fiber, lean proteins, and healthy fats:

FIBER	HEALTHY FATS
Beans	Avocado
Fresh whole fruits (NOT fruit juice!)	Olive Oil
Green Leafy Vegetables	Salmon
Whole grains	Walnut
LEAN PROTEINS	
Free Range Chicken Breast	
Free Range Turkey Breast	
Free Range, Grass Fed Beef	
Wild caught tilapia, tuna, and salmon	

And remember to drink PLENTY of water. Filtered is best, alkaline is even better. You should aim for 50% of your body weight in ounces each day. Work up to it; don't try to do it at one time if you are not otherwise a daily water drinker!

So take this book with you to the grocery store and use this chapter as your very first healthy shopping list! You will be well on your way to a healthier you when you start adding the right foods and drinks to your daily intake and eliminating the wrong ones.

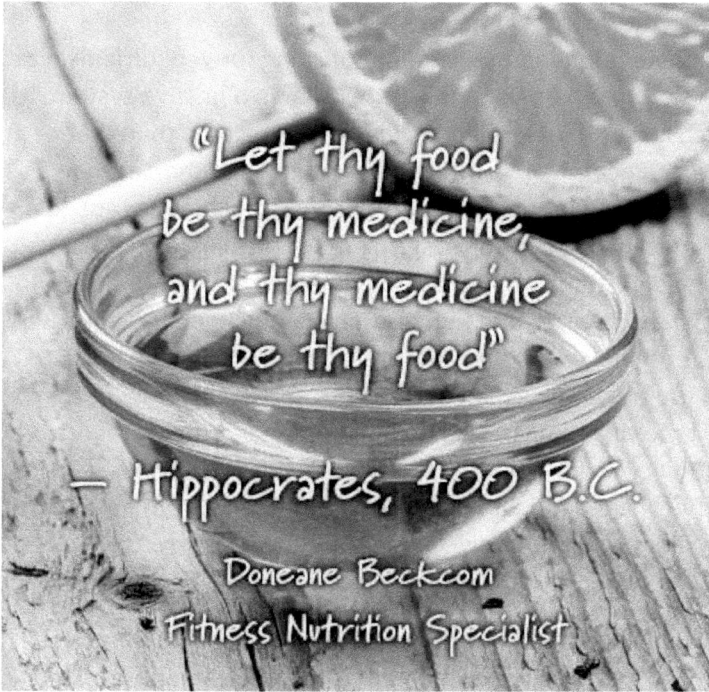

"Let thy food be thy medicine, and thy medicine be thy food"

— Hippocrates, 400 B.C.

Doneane Beckcom
Fitness Nutrition Specialist

When I studied for and tested to become a certified nutritionist, I learned one of my favorite quotes with regard to food: "Let thy food be thy medicine, and thy medicine be thy food." Hippocrates, the father of modern medicine (doctors still take the Hippocratic Oath), said this 400 years before the birth of Jesus. At that time, this was all mankind had for medicine – food, plants, herbs, nuts – whatever had a medicinal value was used to treat illness because that is all there was!

We NEED to return to this mindset. Our bodies were not meant to deal with chemicals, poisons, metals, all the things that can be present in modern-day medicines, drugs, prescriptions – however you categorize them. Our bodies were meant to eat a plant-based diet, not consume large amounts of animal protein and artificial ingredients.

Don't misunderstand me; I am not pushing for vegetarianism or veganism. But when you look at the human digestive system, it is much closer to a herbivore's digestive anatomy than that of a carnivore. A carnivore's intestinal tract is much shorter than a herbivore's or a human's, in part because raw meat needs to move quickly through the system before turning rancid. The average digestion cycle for a carnivore is roughly 6 – 8 hours. In contrast, herbivores and humans have a much longer digestive tract: food moves through it more slowly because breaking down the fibers from plants takes longer and the body needs more time to assimilate the nutrients from it. The average digestion cycle for a herbivore and human is 18 – 24 hours. This is part of the reason why doctors discourage us from eating too much red meat, as our digestive tract is not designed to handle a lot of animal protein, cooked or not!

When I decided to take control and change my eating habits, I wanted to get back to a more natural way of eating. I grabbed every resource I could find to figure out what I needed to do. Books by Dr. Don Colbert are a great resource, easy to read and full of useful information about what to eat, what not to eat, and how to get healthy by using foods and periodic fasting. Check the resources section at the back of this book for more information on his work and other doctors and authors who can help you on your personal journey.

What really spoke to me was the concept of the Mediterranean Diet, in a book by Dr. Colbert "What Would Jesus Eat." This was the very first book I read when I started my nutrition journey, and it was recommended by a good friend. In fact, she gave me hers and said "Keep it!" and then to pass it on to someone else who needs it. In the past 15 years, it has been passed around to many people, and I hope everyone who has had my copy has

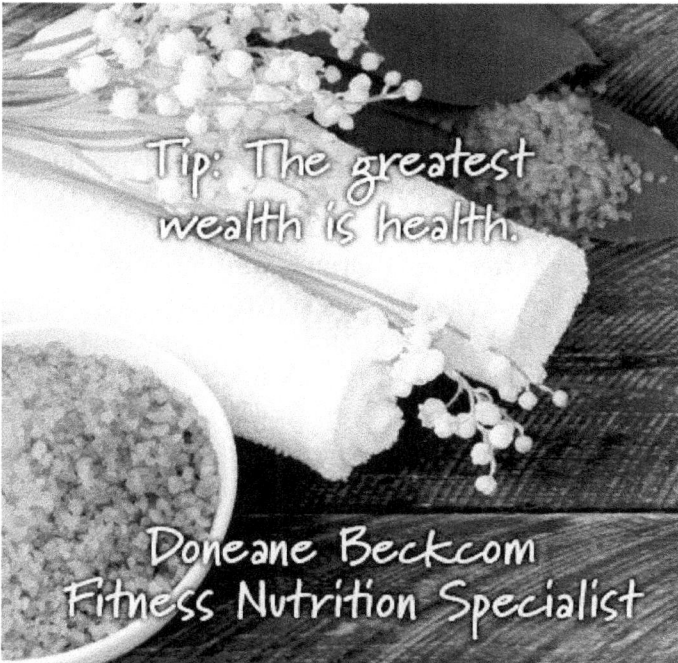

Tip: The greatest wealth is health.

Doneane Beckcom
Fitness Nutrition Specialist

benefitted from it! It is a very easy read, an eye-opener, and I highly recommend it.

Before the industrial age, people ate fish, whole grains, fruits and vegetables, drank lots of water, and walked everywhere they went. And they drank wine! They stayed healthy by the foods they ate and their daily exercise. If someone was sick, the medicine of choice, again, was food, and typically plant-based remedies.

The food industry in the United States scares the heck out of me. Learning what was happening to our food before it got to my table was an eye-opener. How our food is making us sick because of how it is produced, handled, processed, packaged. How our children are maturing physically at an alarmingly younger age now than in the past because of added hormones in animal protein. It is shocking, believe me. The way people ate in ancient times is vastly different from today's diet. How our food is processed now is so different from even a few hundred years ago.

It is important to educate yourself as much as you can about your body and how it works. I encourage you to look at the resource list at the back of this book for some suggestions for other easy reading material that will help you better understand the fascinating machine you are living in! It has been my experience that if a person knows his or her body better, how everything functions together as a whole, then making healthy changes are much easier. And every book or resource you will see at the end of this book I have personally read and 'digested' over the years. They have helped me to get to where I am today with my health, nutrition, and exercise, and I rely on the information in them to help my clients – and you – to make better choices for a long and healthy life.

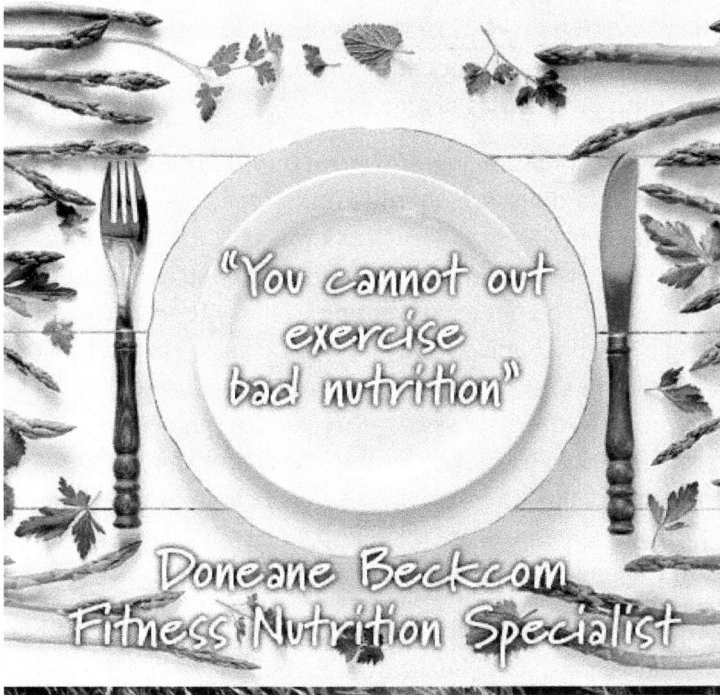

"You cannot out exercise bad nutrition"

Doneane Beckcom
Fitness Nutrition Specialist

It does not matter how much you exercise, how often you do Yoga or attend boot camp class, if you are not getting proper nutrition. If you are putting garbage into your body, you are defeating the purpose of your exercise. A healthy body is not just looking good on the outside; it is being healthy on the inside too.

Now, that's not to say that you can't look good on the outside but still be really unhealthy on the inside. I am living proof of that, or at least I was for many years. The key to really good health starts on the inside.

That is why for years I have called myself the "Personal Trainer for Your Insides." Because that is exactly what I do – I train you to put the right things on the inside so that you become healthier from the inside out. The healthier you are on the inside, the healthier your outsides will be, and that health will spill over into other areas of your life.

Chemicals and unnatural ingredients in our foods are destroying our health. Our bodies are not meant to process things that it does not recognize as food – such as trans fats, artificial ingredients, preservatives – it is just not designed to function that way. But, if you have been eating this way for many years, breaking those old habits is not going to be easy. I am not going to sugar-coat this for you – it will be HARD. It will take dedication, determination, strength, patience, resolve, everything you can muster to have the willingness, and the willpower, to make it happen. Don't worry about motivation – that's where I come in. I will be your biggest cheerleader! But YOU are the one who has to decide to make it happen.

My eating plans revolve around the concept of carb cycling. It is a great way to learn new healthy eating habits, while taking out the unhealthy carbs that most of us eat way too much of, and which may contribute to a lot of the symptoms you may be experiencing. It is also a very healthy way to lose weight. AND, because this is a clean eating plan, it will also help to alleviate your hormonal symptoms as well. It is a win-win situation!

You may have heard of this concept before, with a diet that was popular a few years ago and still comes around every now and then. That particular plan was an extreme version of carb cycling, to the point that people on this diet often became very ill from the adverse side-effects of totally removing ALL carbs from their diet, which is not a good idea. Healthy carbs are responsible for helping our brains produce the "feel good" chemicals, serotonin and dopamine, which help control moods.

Take away all the carbs and most people turn into raving lunatics! Horrible mood swings, brain fog, and the risk of ketosis, which can be dangerous and sometimes fatal.

Here is a list of low carb foods (some may surprise you):

PROTEINS	FRUITS/VEGGIES
Beef	Alfalfa Sprouts
Chicken	Asparagus
Clams	Broccoli
Crab	Cabbage
Duck	Celery
Eggs	Cucumber
Fish	Endive
Lamb	Lemons / Limes
Pork	Lettuce
Shrimp	Mushrooms
Tofu	Olives
Turkey	Onions
Veal	Oregano
	Parsley
	Pickles
	Radishes
	Raspberries / Cranberries
	Seaweed
	Spinach
	Strawberries / Blackberries
	Sweet Peppers

FATS/OILS	CONDIMENTS
Butter	Barbecue Sauce
Cheese	Mayonnaise
Corn Oil	Mustard
Olive Oil	Salad Dressings
Peanut Oil	Sour Cream
Safflower Oil	Soy Sauce
Soybean Oil	Tartar Sauce
Sunflower Oil	Vinegar

And now for the high carbs list (you probably are familiar with these already, but it doesn't hurt to be reminded):

GRAINS	FRUITS
Bagels	Apple
Barley	Apricot
Bran	Banana
Breads	Blueberry
Buckwheat	Dates
Cereals	Fig
Cornmeal	Grapes
Muesli	Orange
Muffins	Pear
Oatmeal	Pineapple
Pasta	Raisins
Shredded wheat	Strawberry
Spaghetti	Watermelon
White rice	
VEGETABLES (HIGH IN STARCHES)	DAIRY
Beans	Chocolate milk
Black eye peas	Low fat, plain yogurt
Carrots	Nonfat milk
Chickpeas	Skim milk
Corn	
Garbanzo beans	
Navy beans	
Peas	
Potatoes	
Refried beans	
Sweet potatoes	
White beans	
OTHER	
Chocolates, Candies, Cookies, Pastries, Table sugar, Cakes, Corn syrup, Fruit juices	

Now, there are some healthy things on this list above; however, if you are trying to lose weight and cut down on carbs (or do a carb cycle program), then this is the list to try and stay away from. They can be added back, in moderation, once you have met your weight loss goal on this type of nutrition plan.

At the end of the book is a link to resources on my webpage where you can learn more about this topic, and also an example of what a Carb Cycle Eating Plan really looks like. I promise you, it is TONS of food and you will not be hungry, but over the course of two cycles, your eating habits will change and you will see a shift in your weight (fat loss and building muscle). It is a great place to start your journey!

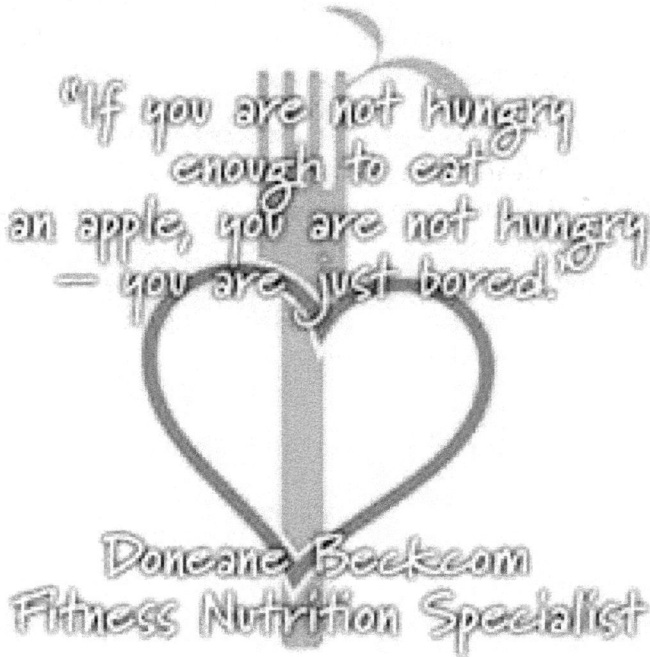

"If you are not hungry enough to eat an apple, you are not hungry — you are just bored."

Doneane Beckcom
Fitness Nutrition Specialist

I eat when I am bored. I admit it. I call it "mindless eating." For the most part when I do this, I eat something healthy; but still, when I am bored the first thing I think about is food. Heaven help me if there are potato chips around when I get bored!

I have had to retrain my brain so that when I feel bored and my mind drifts to the snacks in the kitchen, I need to engage in some activity that is going to stimulate my brain. Play a brain game on my phone, take a break and read a book for a bit, listen to some music, play with my dogs, something that engages my brain and lifts the feeling of boredom.

If you really ARE hungry, then consider whether or not you are hungry enough to eat a medium piece of fruit: an apple, a pear, half-a-cup of berries. If not, you are probably just bored. If you really ARE hungry, then by all means grab something healthy and chow down. But be mindful about it, don't just eat just because, and don't eat just anything!

Which brings me to another subject: eating for comfort. Many of us find comfort in food. Sometimes I do, but if I am really having a difficult emotional time I usually go in the opposite direction and eat nothing. When my hormones are going crazy and I am having cramps or a backache, MAN do I want some greasy fast food or some fried chicken or a corn dog, Oh, the humanity! And when I fall off of the healthy eating wagon and find myself in a fast food drive-through, I do NOT let myself feel guilty! Nope. Because I know this is not a habit and it does not happen very often. Some comfort food might just make me feel better. At least for a few minutes . . .

If needing comfort food is something that occurs multiple times a week, it could be something you need to address. Mindless eating or running to your comfort food can be a sign that you are experiencing depression – maybe your Vitamin B and D levels have gotten low, so your feel good brain chemicals are misfiring. Or maybe there is more to it, and your doctor might need to order some lab tests. So please, if this describes you, make an appointment and get checked out.

If your comfort food/bored/mindless eating is an occasional thing (mine happens once every few months or so if my cycle is particularly rough), then not to worry. Indulge. But get BACK on that wagon tomorrow. I know when I fall off, I feel absolutely HORRIBLE the next day in my gut and sometimes in my head, because the yuck in the fast food I just had to have is wreaking havoc on my otherwise healthy insides, so I WILL pay for it. And I KNOW this. But sometimes the need for that comforting corn dog or greasy fried chicken yells louder than the voice that tells me to always eat healthy!

Bottom line: don't fret over an occasional slip-up when you feel the need to eat something that is not otherwise healthy. Just be aware of this habit, and get it in check if it is happening several times a week. And check yourself before eating: am I really hungry, and if so, am I hungry enough for a piece of fruit? If not, go find something else to do!

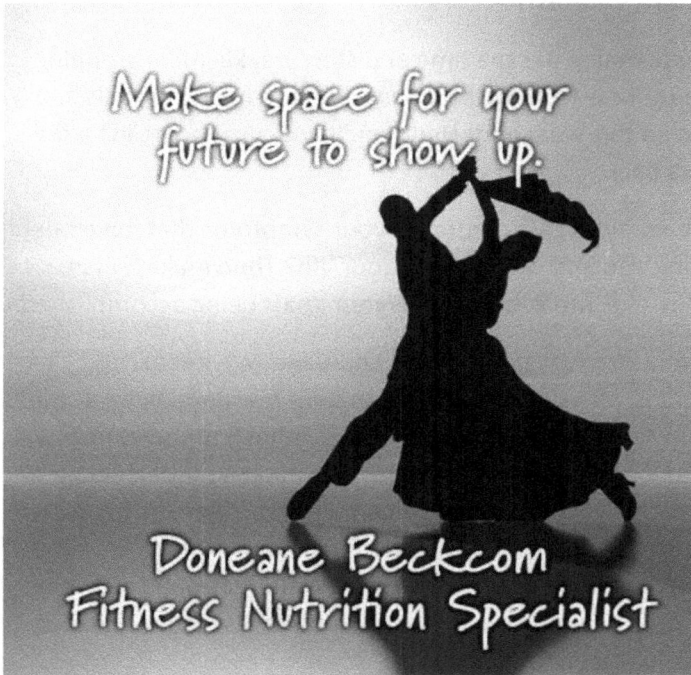

Earlier we talked about doing something now that in the future you would be thankful for. That also includes getting out of the way so that the future can happen.

If you set your mind to accomplish a goal, why step in the way and obstruct it?

Are you making plans to lose weight, but your kitchen still contains all sorts of junk food? Get that stuff out of the way and make room for the healthy you of the future to show up!

Are you planning to start a new exercise routine? Then set aside your personal time to accomplish this each day, and let your family and friends know that this is your "golden time." You are

NOT to be disturbed! And do not let anything get in the way – don't make excuses!

Are you planning to save time and start weekly meal prepping? Then learn how to shop, cook, and prepare healthy meals and get started this weekend! Hint: you'll find a shopping list a few chapters back.

Are you ready to gain control of your symptoms that have been bothering you and interrupting your life? Then make a plan, stick to it, execute it, and watch your goals being accomplished.

Some of us are very good at self-sabotage. We get excited, make grand plans, and follow them for a few days, even a week, and then something happens: we stop following them. I know. I have done it! I will set a course for action on a new schedule to get up early, work out, have some quiet time, get stuff done before work, and inevitably something happens and I get off course. And then we make excuses. "Well, I can start over next week," or "I needed that extra hour of sleep because I did not sleep well." You know the drill.

When I decided years ago to change my habits and get healthy again, I had to get out of the way. It was almost as if I was directing myself from someone else's body and brain, making myself do things that were foreign, uncomfortable, and challenging. It was not easy, and it took a long time. But once I replaced the bad habits with good ones and started to see and FEEL a difference, it was EASY to get out of the way of that progress!

You have to be READY. No one can do this for you.

I will give you an example from a recent client. Peggy (not her real name) had all sorts of health problems which were attributed almost 100% to the fact that she was addicted to food: she was morbidly obese. She had bariatric surgery three

70

years before I met her, and she lost 85 pounds. But she did not get any follow-up care or counseling to address the underlying cause: she was addicted to food. Like a lot of patients who have bariatric surgery and fail to get aftercare to deal with the psychological issues underlying their obesity, Peggy figured out a way to "get around" her surgical intervention, and she started eating more and more, and eating unhealthily again. She gained the 85 pounds back, and more, and she started having health issues not present before the surgery. I ran into her at the grocery store one day, and while we were talking I could tell she felt guilty about the things in her basket. She tried to explain why she had them. I just smiled and said I understood, but to let me know when she was ready to make a change. Over the course of several months, I would see that she signed up for different free eBooks I offered on my website about strategies for healthy eating, and she would get excited about this or that new plan she was going to try. But then, when her plans did not pan out, she went back to her old ways again. Finally, with additional uncomfortable health problems developing, she went back to her doctors and got a complete check-up to find out what was wrong. Once she was diagnosed with additional health issues, she was scared into taking the steps she needed to take back her life and deal with her food addiction. No amount of me telling her what she needed to do, or her husband begging her to get help, or her friends or other family members trying to help, was going to make Peggy do what she needed to do. She had to get out of the way and do what she KNEW she had to do – deal with her food addiction or die. And she is doing it slowly, to ensure that her bad habits are replaced by healthy ones that will last for the rest of her life. I am happy to say that just before this book went to print, she was on track and had lost a few pounds, which made her feel good about herself again and the possibility that she really COULD do it!

Does Peggy's story sound like yours? Maybe you have not gone the surgical route, but you were once healthy and you are now trying to get back on track? Have you tried to get on a plan but just keep slipping back into your old ways? Are you frustrated, tired, feel bad and depressed? You NEED the support of a group of people who are like-minded and want the same thing: good health for the rest of your life!

Think about it . . . when was the last time you set a course for some plan – health, work, or a personal goal – worked the plan, and saw some results? It felt GREAT, right? That is what I want you to work toward, taking small steps, one at a time. Those all-or-nothing plans do not work with most people. Small, achievable goals which can be felt, seen, and measured are the ones that will create lasting results.

For help and motivation, check out the resources at the end of the book, or join my Facebook group to get daily motivation from ME. I will be your biggest cheerleader to help YOU get out of the way and reach your goals. Can you get out of your own way today and take those first steps toward your health goals?

EPILOGUE: LIFE IS BEAUTIFUL AGAIN!

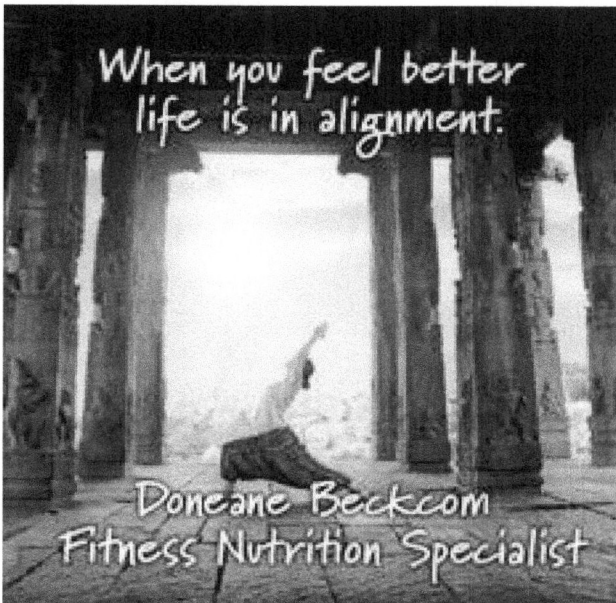

When you feel better life is in alignment.

Doneane Beckcom
Fitness Nutrition Specialist

What a great feeling it is to finally feel better, and to know that it happened because you took control and decided it was time to make healthy changes. I want you to be able to identify with this statement in your future!

I can still remember when I was not feeling well, eating badly, and not taking care of my body. Because I let it go on for so long, feeling bad actually felt normal to me. Waking up each day stiff and sore, having trouble breathing, being in pain, seemed normal then. When I came out of that fog and realized how good I could feel, it was amazing!

What is really amazing is that when you feel better, life becomes clearer. Chaos begins to disappear, things align as they should, freedom and joy are attainable, and often every day occurrences. Feeling better physically is the key to feeling better emotionally, psychologically, and spiritually. And when all those things fall into place, your decision-making will also be clearer, cleaner, and less chaotic.

Life really can be beautiful in so many ways. But the BEST way is when you are enjoying life fully because you FEEL good, and you got there by making the decision to make healthy changes in your life and stick to them. Let today be THE day that your journey begins. Use the resources in this book as a guide and let me help you say – and believe – "My life is beautiful!"

Doneane

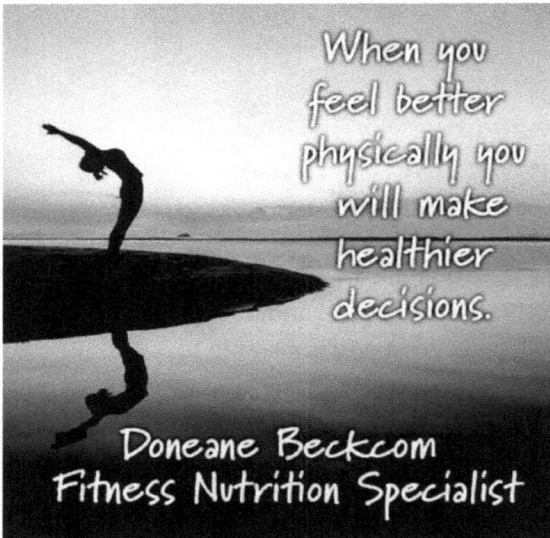

When you feel better physically you will make healthier decisions.

Doneane Beckcom
Fitness Nutrition Specialist

RESOURCES

Don Colbert, MD

What Would Jesus Eat? Siloam 2005

What You Don't Know May Be Killing You: Siloam 2000

Living in Divine Health: Siloam 2005

The Seven Pillars of Health: Siloam 2007

Eat This and Live: Siloam 2009

Toxic Relief: Siloam 2001

Dr. Mehmet C. Oz and Dr. Michael F. Roizen

YOU the Owner's Manual: Scribner 2005

YOU Staying Young: Scribner 2007

Dr. John R. Lee

What Your Doctor May Not be Telling You about Menopause: Warner Books 1996

T. Colin Campbell, PhD and Thomas M. Campbell, PhD

The China Study: BenBella Books 2005

Jonny Bowden

The 150 Healthiest Foods on Earth: Fair Winds Press 2007

Gene Stone and T. Colin Campbell, PhD

Forks over Knives: The Experiment LLC 2001

David Zinczenko and Matt Goulding

Eat This Not That: Rodale 2008

Dr. Joel Fuhrman

Eat to Live Cookbook: Harper Collins 2013

YOGA RESOURCES

Anything and everything by Rodney Yee. He was my go-to instructor when I first started out and his books, flash cards, and DVDs are all excellent and easy to follow for beginners as well as more advanced students. All of his products are available on Amazon.

Carb Cycle Sample Meal Plans

This is a snap-shot of what the Carb Cycle Eating Plan looks like. This is just one shopping list and one day's meals. (To show how EASY it is and how MUCH food is on this plan!) Each cycle lasts for two weeks, and then a new cycle with different foods added starts, for a total of four two-week cycles. In eight weeks you will see changed habits and weight loss (most likely, but everyone's results are different).

14 DAY CARB CYCLE; SAMPLE CYCLE 1

FOODS TO CHOOSE FROM:

Fish: Salmon, Sole, Flounder, Tilapia, Canned Tuna (in water) (wild caught is best!)

Poultry: Chicken breast, Turkey breast, Ground lean turkey, Eggs (2 eggs = 1 serving), Egg whites (4 egg whites = 1 serving)

Vegetables: Artichoke, Asparagus, Bell peppers (all colors), Broccoli, Brussels sprouts, Cabbage, Carrots, Cauliflower, Celery, Cucumber, Eggplant, Garlic, Green Beans, Green leafy veggies (like turnip greens, mustard greens, kale), Leeks, Lettuce (all varieties), Mushrooms, Okra, Onions, Parsley, Scallions, Spinach, Tomatoes, Watercress

Low Sugar Fruit (2 servings per day): Apples, Berries (all types), Grapefruit (unless you take a statin drug), Oranges, Peaches, Pears, Plums, Prickly Pear Cactus, Prunes, Red Grapes

Probiotic Foods (2 servings per day): Yogurt (low fat, plain), Kefir, Low fat acidophilus milk, Cottage cheese with live active cultures, Tempeh, Sauerkraut, Kimchi

Healthy Fats (1 to 2 tablespoons per day): Fish Oil supplement, Olive Oil, Flaxseed Oil

SAMPLE MENUS

FIRST DRINK OF THE MORNING:
8 oz. cup of hot water with the juice of one medium lemon

BREAKFAST CHOICES:
1. 2 scrambled egg whites prepared with NO oil, ½ grapefruit or other fruit, 1 cup green tea
2. 6 oz. Fat-free plain yogurt with 1 cup berries or other fruit, 1 cup green tea
3. 2 hard boiled or poached eggs, ½ grapefruit or other fruit, 1 cup green tea
4. Yogurt smoothie, 1 cup green tea
5. Low-fat or fat-free cottage cheese with live active cultures, 1 serving fruit, 1 cup green tea

SNACK CHOICES:
1. 6 oz. Fat free plain yogurt mixed with 1 to 2 tablespoons fresh fruit
2. 1 serving of fruit
3. 1 cup fresh berries
4. Yogurt smoothie
5. Raw vegetables and 1 tablespoon low-fat or fat-free vegetable dip

LUNCH CHOICES:
1. Large green salad topped with tuna and 1 tablespoon olive oil and 2 tablespoons balsamic vinegar, 1 cup green tea

2. Large green salad with loads of vegetables, 1 cup green tea
3. Large bowl of low sodium chicken vegetable soup with NO pasta or potatoes, 1 cup green tea
4. Baby spinach salad with tomatoes and crumble low-fat Feta cheese, 1 cup green tea
5. Lettuce wraps with grilled chicken, tossed salad, 1 cup green tea

DINNER CHOICES:
1. Grilled chicken or fish, unlimited amounts of vegetables (steamed or raw), 1 cup green tea
2. Eggplant Parmesan made with low-fat Parmesan cheese, unlimited cleansing vegetables, 1 cup green tea
3. Ground turkey patties, Side salad, 1 cup green tea
4. Stir fry vegetables in 1 tablespoon olive oil, add garlic powder and lite soy sauce, 1 cup green tea

SOCIAL MEDIA LINKS

Email: 1NutritionExpert@gmail.com

Website: www.fitnessnutritionconsulting.com

Facebook Page:
https://www.facebook.com/fitnessnutritionconsulting/

Facebook Group:
https://www.facebook.com/groups/612753335548533/

Twitter: https://twitter.com/doneanebeckcom

YouTube Channel:
https://www.youtube.com/channel/UCfTa5NafjU2b71fHhxqA3
0A

Pinterest: https://www.pinterest.com/dbeckcom/

Bold Radio: Join Doneane every Tuesday at 1 PM Eastern for her live internet radio show "Hot Mamas: Living Better at Any Age" at http://www.boldradiostation.com

Women's Broadcast Television Network: Join Doneane on the WBTVN for her show "Fit & Healthy After 50 with Doneane" which airs monthly. Check out her show and other videos on her station page at http://wbtvn.tv/host/doneane-beckcom/

www.ingramcontent.com/pod-product-compliance
Lightning Source LLC
Chambersburg PA
CBHW070909280326
41934CB00008B/1644